# Introduction to Supportive Psychotherapy

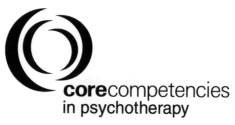

**core**competencies
in psychotherapy

*Glen O. Gabbard, M.D., Series Editor*

# Introduction to Supportive Psychotherapy

## Arnold Winston, M.D.
Chairman, Department of Psychiatry and Behavioral Sciences,
Beth Israel Medical Center, New York, New York
Professor and Vice Chairman, Department of Psychiatry and
Behavioral Sciences, Albert Einstein College of Medicine,
Bronx, New York

## Richard N. Rosenthal, M.D.
Chairman, Department of Psychiatry,
St. Luke's–Roosevelt Hospital Center, New York, New York
Professor of Clinical Psychiatry, Department of Psychiatry,
Columbia University College of Physicians and Surgeons,
New York, New York

## Henry Pinsker, M.D.
Honorary Attending, Department of Psychiatry and Behavioral Sciences,
Beth Israel Medical Center, New York, New York
Clinical Professor of Psychiatry (retired), Department of Psychiatry,
Mount Sinai School of Medicine, New York, New York

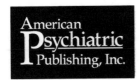

American Psychiatric Publishing, Inc.

Washington, DC
London, England

Copyright © 2004 American Psychiatric Publishing, Inc.
ALL RIGHTS RESERVED

Some material in this book is adapted from Pinsker H: *A Primer of Supportive Psychotherapy*. Hillsdale, NJ, The Analytic Press, 1997; and Winston A, Winston B: *Handbook of Integrated Short-Term Psychotherapy*. Washington, DC, American Psychiatric Publishing, 2002.

Manufactured in the United States of America on acid-free paper
08  07  06  05        5  4  3  2
First Edition

Typeset in Adobe's Berling Roman and Frutiger

American Psychiatric Publishing, Inc.
1000 Wilson Boulevard
Arlington, VA 22209-3901
www.appi.org

**Library of Congress Cataloging-in-Publication Data**
Winston, Arnold, 1935–
    Introduction to supportive psychotherapy / Arnold Winston, Richard N. Rosenthal, Henry Pinsker.—1st ed.
        p. ; cm. – (Core competencies in psychotherapy)
    Includes bibliographical references and index.
    ISBN 1-58562-147-1 (pbk. : alk. paper)
    1. Supportive psychotherapy. 2. Psychotherapist and patient. I. Rosenthal, Richard N. II. Pinsker, Henry, 1928– III. Title. IV. Series.
    [DNLM: 1. Psychotherapy–methods. 2. Professional-Patient Relations. 3. Psychotherapeutic Processes. WM 420 W783i 2004]
    RC489.S86W55 2004
    616.89'14–dc22

                                                                2003065592

**British Library Cataloguing in Publication Data**
A CIP record is available from the British Library.

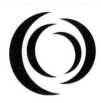

# Contents

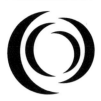

# Introduction to the Core Competencies in Psychotherapy Series

**W**ith the extraordinary progress in the neurosciences and psychophar-macology in recent years, some psychiatric training programs have de-emphasized psychotherapy education. Many residents and educators have decried the loss of the "mind" in the increasing emphasis on the bio-logical basis of mental illness and the shift toward somatic treatments as the central therapeutic strategy in psychiatry. This shift in emphasis has been compounded by the common practice in our managed care era of "split treatment," meaning that psychiatrists are often relegated to seeing the patient for a brief medication management session, while the psychother-apy is conducted by a mental health professional from another discipline. This shift in emphasis has created considerable concern among both psy-chiatric educators and the consumers of psychiatric education—the resi-dents themselves.

The importance of psychotherapy in the training of psychiatrists has re-cently been reaffirmed, however, as a result of the widespread movement toward the establishment of core competencies throughout all medical specialties. In 1999 both the Accreditation Council for Graduate Medical Education (ACGME) and the American Board of Medical Specialties (ABMS) recognized that a set of organizing principles was necessary to measure competence in medical education. These six principles—patient care, medical knowledge, interpersonal and communication skills, practice-based learning and improvement, professionalism, and systems-based practice—are now collectively referred to as the *core competencies* in medical education.

This movement within medical education was a direct consequence of a broader movement launched by the U.S. Department of Education approximately 20 years ago. All educational projects, including those involving accreditation, had to develop outcome measures. Those entrusted with the training of physicians were no exception.

Like all medical specialties, psychiatry has risen to the occasion by making attempts to translate the notion of core competencies into meaningful psychiatric terms. The inherent ambiguity of a term like "competence" has sparked much discussion among psychiatric educators. Does the term mean that practitioners are sufficiently skilled that one would refer a family member to them for treatment without hesitation? Or does the term imply rudimentary knowledge and practice that would ensure a reasonable degree of safety? These questions are not yet fully resolved. The basic understanding of what is meant by core competencies will be evolving over the next few years as various groups within medicine and psychiatry strive to articulate reasonable standards for educators.

As of July 2002, the Psychiatry Residency Review Committee (RRC) mandated that all psychiatric residency training programs must begin implementing the six core competencies in clinical and didactic curricula. Those programs that fail to do so may receive citations when they undergo accreditation surveys. This mandate also requires training directors to develop more sophisticated means of evaluating the progress and learning of residents in their programs.

As part of the process of adapting the core competencies to psychiatry, the Psychiatry RRC felt that reasonable competence in five different forms of psychotherapy—long-term psychodynamic psychotherapy, supportive psychotherapy, cognitive behavioral psychotherapy, brief psychotherapy, and psychotherapy combined with psychopharmacology—should be an outcome of a good psychiatric education for all psychiatric residents.

Many training programs have had to scramble to find faculty who are well trained in these modalities and teaching materials to facilitate the learning process. American Psychiatric Publishing, Inc., felt that the publication of basic texts in each of the five mandated areas would be of great value to training programs. So in 2002 Dr. Robert Hales, editor-in-chief at American Psychiatric Publishing, appointed me to be the series editor of a new line of five books. This series is titled Core Competencies in Psychotherapy and features five brief texts by leading experts in each of the psychotherapies. Each volume covers the key principles of practice in the treatment and also suggests ways to evaluate whether residents have been trained to a level of competence in each of the therapies. (For more information about the books in this series and their availability, please visit www.appi.org.)

True expertise in psychotherapy requires many years of experience with skilled supervision and consultation. However, the basic tools can be learned during residency training so that freshly minted psychiatrists are prepared to deliver necessary treatments to the broad range of patients they encounter.

These books will be valuable adjuncts to the traditional methods of psychotherapy education: supervision, classroom teaching, and clinical experience with a variety of patients. We feel confident that mastery of the material in these five volumes will constitute a major step in the acquisition of competency in psychotherapy and, ultimately, the compassionate care of patients who come to us for help.

*Glen O. Gabbard, M.D., Series Editor*
Brown Foundation Chair of Psychoanalysis
Professor of Psychiatry
Director of Psychotherapy Education
Director, Baylor Psychiatry Clinic
Baylor College of Medicine
Houston, Texas

# Introduction

The Residency Review Committee for Psychiatry has mandated that all psychiatry residents achieve competence in five types of psychotherapy. In this book, we outline a systematic approach to one of these therapies: supportive psychotherapy.

This book is directed at beginning therapists who need to learn the fundamentals of psychotherapy and, in particular, how to talk with psychotherapy patients. All practitioners search for effective ways to treat patients. We believe that the beginning resident attempting to practice supportive psychotherapy needs clear guidelines for the conduct and progression of psychotherapy from beginning to end. Accordingly, we have attempted to present clear guidelines to help the beginner in four major areas: maintaining a positive therapeutic alliance, understanding and formulating patients' problems, setting realistic treatment goals, and knowing what to say to patients (technique).

We begin with the basic principles of supportive psychotherapy and the position of supportive psychotherapy on a continuum from supportive to expressive psychotherapy, based on the extent and level of a patient's psychopathology. We describe supportive psychotherapy interventions available to the therapist, how to perform a thorough patient evaluation and case formulation, and the process of setting realistic goals with the patient.

Evidence for the efficacy of supportive psychotherapy is presented with a summary of a number of outcome trials. The general framework of supportive psychotherapy—including indications, phases of treatment, initiation and termination of sessions, and professional boundaries—are outlined. We include therapeutic relationship issues (transference, countertransference, therapeutic alliance) and self-disclosure guidelines.

There is a chapter on crisis intervention, which uses many supportive psychotherapy approaches, and one on special populations, including the chronically mentally ill and patients with comorbid conditions. We conclude with a discussion of how to determine whether a psychiatry resident has achieved competence in supportive psychotherapy.

## Acknowledgments

We are indebted to a number of colleagues for their help in supplying material for this book and help during its writing. We owe particular thanks to Mimi Lee for her help in preparing the manuscript. Beverly Winston provided important feedback on each of the chapters.

We wish to acknowledge the importance of the Beth Israel Brief Psychotherapy Research Program in providing the milieu for the writing of this book and our colleagues from this program, especially John Christopher Muran, Jeremy Safran, and Lisa Wallner Samstag. Finally, we are grateful to the Supportive Psychotherapy Study Group for help in developing many of the ideas contained in this book, including Victor Goldin, Esther Goldman, David Hellerstein, David Janeway, Steve Klee, Lee Shomstein, Fran Silverman, Jeffrey Solgan, Adam Wilensky, and Philip Yanowitch.

*Arnold Winston, M.D.*
*Richard N. Rosenthal, M.D.*
*Henry Pinsker, M.D.*

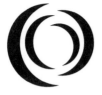

# Basic Principles of Supportive Psychotherapy

## Origins

The concept of supportive psychotherapy was developed early in the twentieth century to describe a treatment approach with objectives more limited than the objectives of psychoanalysis. The objective of supportive treatment was not to change the patient's personality but to help the patient cope with symptoms in order to prevent relapse of serious mental illness or, in the case of a relatively healthy person, to help him or her deal with a transient problem. A dictionary definition of *support* says it well: "to bear the weight of," "to keep from falling," and "to keep from weakening or failing; to strengthen" (*The American Heritage Dictionary of the English Language*, 4th edition).

Various definitions of *supportive psychotherapy* have been organized around 1) the therapist's objectives—to maintain or improve the patient's self-esteem, to minimize or prevent recurrence of symptoms, and to maximize the patient's adaptive capacities (American Association of Directors of Psychiatric Residency Training 2003); 2) the patient's goals—"to maintain or reestablish the best-possible level of functioning given the limitations of his or her personality, native ability, and life circumstances" (Ursano and Silberman 1999); or 3) what supportive psychotherapy is not—that is, an explanation of what elements of expressive therapy have been subtracted, as illustrated in Dewald's pioneering theoretical presentation (Dewald 1964, 1971).

Defined narrowly, as in earlier years, supportive psychotherapy is a body of techniques, such as advice, exhortation, and encouragement, used to treat severely impaired patients. In practice, supportive psychotherapy provided by trained psychotherapists was invariably embedded in psychodynamic understanding. Defined broadly, as has been the trend, supportive psychotherapy is an approach with wide applicability; it is the most widely practiced form of individual psychotherapy. The narrow definition was based on theory; the broad definition evolved because authors who wrote about supportive psychotherapy described and explained their conversations with patients.

In the first half of the twentieth century, psychoanalysis was essentially the only formal psychological treatment. Treatment that was less sophisticated than psychoanalysis was denigrated and referred to as *suggestion*, an approach that had been used with occasional success as a treatment for hysteria, the object of Freud's earliest attention. Interactions between physician and patient that were not psychoanalysis soon became known as psychotherapy, and it was evident that there was a lot more to this therapy than mere suggestion.

Starting with hypotheses about the causes of symptoms and personality problems, psychoanalytic thinkers ultimately created a general theory of mental organization and behavior that is generally referred to as psychodynamic theory. Many concepts of psychodynamic theory have become so widely disseminated that they are now accepted by the educated public as established truth about mental life; some concepts have vanished. Psychoanalysis, which was invented as a treatment for patients with clear-cut symptoms, evolved to become a treatment intended to produce lasting personality change in well-integrated, intelligent individuals.

Therapy with less ambitious goals became known as psychodynamic psychotherapy. At various times, it has been called psychoanalytically oriented psychotherapy, intensive psychotherapy, uncovering psychotherapy, change-oriented psychotherapy, and insight-directed psychotherapy. Psychodynamic psychotherapy became the most widely practiced psychological treatment approach in the United States. It was taught as the embodiment of theories of personality development, and it invariably presented a treatment model with the objectives of reversing the primary disease process or restructuring the personality (Ursano and Silberman 1999). Teaching based on long-term models has provided little guidance about what to talk about with the patient who is seen once a month in a medication clinic.

Psychoanalysis and psychotherapy were originally seen as treatments for neurosis, which was the principle concern of office-based (i.e., non-hospital) psychiatrists. Neurosis was conceptualized as an unconscious attempt to solve a psychological conflict. As psychotherapy became more widely accepted, therapists found themselves responsible for a broader range of clinical problems, such as major mental disorder, personality disorder, and substance abuse, all of which were outside the scope of the primordial psychotherapy. Further, because of practical considerations (including payment), treatment often consisted of a small number of visits, with goals limited to the presenting problem. Flexible response to clinical reality called for more general use of supportive approaches, although some clinicians struggled with the thought that they were diluting the "real" psychotherapy. In fact, they were applying a different psychotherapy. Research studies support the clinical observations that brief and supportive therapies are effective for a broad range of conditions (Conte 1994; Winston and Winston 2002).

The usual approach to the education of psychotherapists has been to teach principles of personality development and symptom formation that have been derived from psychoanalysis. Techniques with specific rationale in psychoanalysis were unfortunately presented as universal techniques required for all psychotherapy. Examples include prolonged silent waiting if the patient stops talking, avoiding direct answers to questions, and ending every meeting with "That's all our time." Supportive psychotherapy, "the Cinderella of psychotherapies" (Sullivan 1971), has for decades been the treatment provided to "the vast majority of patients seen in psychiatric clinics and mental health centers" (Werman 1984, p. ix), where inexperienced therapists are most likely to be found. It was assumed that the student would automatically know how to provide treatment that was thought to be less sophisticated than the model that had been taught. Some trainees with innate interpersonal skills and empathy were effective from the start. Most figured out how to do it as they matured in practice, but for the most part, they did not conceptualize the rationale for what they did and thus could not teach it. Some therapists engaged in an irrational, unintegrated mixture of expressive and supportive approaches—for example, encouraging the patient to talk about his or her past without a plan for use of the material; or providing concrete assistance without encouraging the patient to master new skills for improving his or her circumstances. As Werman (1984) observed, "the patient and therapist may continue their meetings for an inordinately long time under the illusion that ongoing insight-oriented psychotherapy is actually taking place, when in fact patient and therapist are merely playing a charade" (p. 12).

## Definition

Supportive psychotherapy is a dyadic treatment that uses direct measures to ameliorate symptoms and maintain, restore, or improve self-esteem, ego function, and adaptive skills. To accomplish these objectives, treatment may involve examination of relationships, real or transferential, and examination of both past and current patterns of emotional response or behavior. *Self-esteem* involves the patient's sense of efficacy, confidence, hope, and self-regard. *Ego functions* include relation to reality, thinking, defense formation, regulation of affect, synthetic function, and others, as enumerated by Beres (1956), Bellak (1958), and other authors. (Ego functions could alternatively be called psychological functions, because they are addressed by behavior therapists and cognitive therapists whose formulations do not include the ego as a component of a mental apparatus. Ego functions are often categorized as "psychic structure.") *Adaptive skills* are actions associated with effective functioning, although the boundary between ego functions and adaptive skills is not sharply defined. The patient's assessment of events is an ego function; the action he or she takes in response to the assessment is an adaptive skill.

In settings other than formal psychotherapy, the term *supportive therapy* may mean nothing more than expression of interest, attention to concrete services, encouragement, and optimism. Such expression is a *supportive relationship* or *supportive contact*, not supportive psychotherapy. To clarify, supportive psychotherapy is based on diagnostic evaluation; the therapist's actions are deliberate and are designed to achieve specified objectives. However, supportive contacts and supportive relationships that do not qualify as psychotherapy may indeed be useful and sustaining. Relationships with family, friends, co-workers, and neighbors may entail much of what is described as supportive psychotherapy. In a study involving college students seeking counseling, those assigned to English professors did as well as those assigned to professional therapists (Strupp and Hadley 1979).

The professional psychotherapeutic relationship, however, is unique. It is not based on reciprocal equality. It exists solely to meet the needs of the patient or client. The therapist's gratification must come from doing the job well, not from the patient's expressions of gratitude and not from using the patient as an audience. In everyday life, there are many motivations for being supportive. In the professional supportive relationship, the motivation must be to meet the patient's needs.

In the psychiatric literature, the terms *supportive therapy* and *supportive psychotherapy* have been used interchangeably. Such interchangeability is unfortunate because the nonspecific support provided to patients with medical or surgical problems is also characterized as supportive therapy. In this book, we use the long form—*supportive psychotherapy*—to emphasize that we are writing about a professional service that is provided in a mental health context by a person trained in mental health theory and practices.

## The Psychotherapy Continuum

Individual psychotherapies are conceptualized as a spectrum or continuum that extends from supportive psychotherapy to psychoanalysis, as shown in Figure 1–1. (Some would place counseling to the left of supportive psychotherapy). From left to right, the continuum begins with supportive psychotherapy, traverses supportive-expressive psychotherapy, expressive-supportive psychotherapy, and finally extends to psychoanalysis. The term *expressive therapy* has been used as a collective term for a variety of approaches that seek personality change through analysis of the relationship between therapist and patient and through development of insight into previously unrecognized feelings, thoughts, needs, and conflicts, following which the patient attempts to consciously resolve and better integrate such conflicts. "As one approaches the midpoint of this spectrum, the distinctions become blurred and less well differentiated. And even the most exploratory and expressive forms of therapy include some supportive components and experiences; and supportive forms of psychotherapy may include an expansion of patients' awareness of their own mental processes, and thus involve elements of exploratory techniques" (Dewald 1994, p. 505). The treatment of most patients involves both supportive and expressive elements, which must be used in a coherent, integrated fashion.

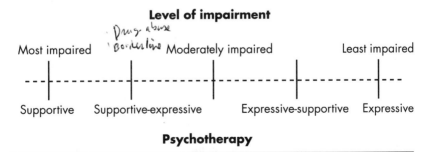

**Figure 1–1.** Impairment/psychotherapy continuum.

Does not
make
sense

Note that the continuum is supportive versus expressive psychotherapy, not supportive psychotherapy versus psychodynamic therapy. In fact, supportive psychotherapy is one of the psychodynamic therapies. Rockland (1989) proposed changing "supportive psychotherapy" as the name of the approach to "psychodynamically oriented supportive therapy," with the acronym *POST*. The term has not become popular, but it reflects the thinking of the profession. In light of the broad definition of *supportive psychotherapy* used by most recent authors, what has often been described as *supportive-expressive therapy* is what most experts on supportive psychotherapy describe as their practice.

## The Psychopathology Continuum

In most clinics, supportive-expressive psychotherapy is the modality indicated for most patients. Who are the patients at the extreme end of the continuum—those who require "pure" supportive psychotherapy—and for whom the therapist's primary concern is amelioration of symptoms or prevention of relapse of major illness? These patients may have significant impairment of psychic structure or ego functions (i.e., they are not defenses), such as cognitive abilities, reality testing, thought process, the capacity to organize behavior, affective regulation, and the capacity to make relational contact with other people. These patients may have disorganized behavior, disorganized thinking, impaired ability to form relationships, and difficulty initiating activity. Causes of the impairment include major mental disorders, pervasive developmental disorder, severe borderline personality disorder, limited intelligence, and limited education or socialization. In meetings with this type of patient, the therapist focuses on the patient's daily activities, medications, and use of resources for social rehabilitation.

At the other end of the spectrum or continuum are individuals who are intact, think clearly and realistically, have at least average intelligence, have accurate perceptions, lead productive lives, and are able to form relationships and to enjoy a wide range of activities relatively free of conflict. These individuals may seek treatment because of self-destructive patterns in interpersonal relationships or because of failure to meet expected personal or employment goals. They may have obsessional, dependent, or avoidant personality disorders; dysthymia; panic disorder; or adjustment disorders. In the middle of the continuum are people with conditions such as narcissistic personality disorder or nonpsychotic depressions. Substance abuse problems occur across the continuum (Winston and Winston 2002).

The most impaired patients require direct interventions aimed at improving ego function, day-to-day coping, and self-esteem. Psychotherapy that is primarily expressive is not possible with these patients. The fact that a patient has the resources and psychological characteristics necessary for expressive therapy does not mean, however, that expressive therapy is indicated. As Hellerstein et al. (1994) pointed out, a strong case can be made for using the supportive model (i.e., supportive-expressive psychotherapy) for most patients, shifting to more expressive measures only as required. Treatment planning always must involve consideration of what the patient wants to accomplish.

## Underlying Assumptions

Supportive psychotherapy relies on *direct measures*. It is not assumed that improvement will develop as a by-product of gaining insight. A major tenet of psychoanalytic psychotherapy was that the unconscious conflict that produced the symptom would become conscious and be worked through and that the symptom would disappear because it was no longer psychologically necessary. In supportive psychotherapy, conscious problems or conflicts are addressed; however, underlying unconscious conflicts and personality distortions are not (Dewald 1964, 1971). Expressive psychotherapy is in fact inherently supportive, but support is an epiphenomenon.

From the point of view of psychoanalytic theory, the patient's defenses are what supportive psychotherapy supports. When therapy is primarily expressive, defenses are identified and examined to determine the underlying conflicts that made defenses necessary. In supportive psychotherapy, defenses are questioned only when they are maladaptive. For example, denial as a strategy for not thinking about the inevitably fatal outcome of one's own life is adaptive, whereas denial that leads to refusal of potentially safe and beneficial treatment is maladaptive. Compulsive habits are maladaptive when they are so rigid that they cause major interference with work or relationships, but compulsive habits can be useful in progressing through graduate education. Passive-aggressive behavior might be explored in expressive psychotherapy as an indicator of unconscious hostility and a need to control others; however, in supportive psychotherapy, the same behavior might be seen as practical and adaptive.

From the supportive vantage point, the relationship between patient and therapist is a relationship between two adults with a common purpose. One provides a service that the other needs, similar in most respects to all other professional relationships. The professional person, the therapist, owes the patient or client respect, full attention, honesty, and vigorous efforts to accomplish the stated purpose by using the knowledge and skills of the profession. Adhering to this discipline is known as staying within boundaries. The interaction may be friendly, but the two individuals do not become friends. The patient may need love; the therapist does not become a lover. The therapist does not help the sexually naive patient by offering sexual contact. The therapist does not advise the patient how to vote, where to vacation, or how to decorate the home; these are products of his or her private, not professional, opinion. The therapist does not seek assistance from the patient. If the therapist finds himself or herself talking at length, giving his or her own experiences, the therapist must determine whether he or she is doing this for the patient's benefit or because the therapist enjoys talking. To use the patient for the latter purpose is exploitation.

In expressive therapy, the relationship between patient and therapist is unlike that in any other relationship. In expressive therapy, the therapist tries to maintain neutrality, minimizing his or her own individual responses so that when the patient describes his or her perceptions of or feelings about the therapist, these can be analyzed as products of projection onto the therapist of the feelings the patient has or had about important figures in current and past life. This redirection of feelings is called transference.

In expressive therapy, analysis of the transference is a key element of the process of understanding the patient's inner life. Because expressive psychotherapy uses analysis of transference to develop understanding of the emotional significance of both past and current relationships, the therapist avoids responses that might gratify the patient's dependency needs, and the therapist tries to minimize the extent to which the patient perceives him or her as a person with opinions, tastes, family, or even personality. It is this technical maneuver that gave rise to the image of the psychotherapist as an individual who parries all questions with evasive answers or with questions back to the patient.

One of the essential differences between supportive psychotherapy and expressive psychotherapies is that in supportive psychotherapy, transference is not ordinarily on the table for discussion. In supportive psychotherapy, transference occurs, as it does in any relationship. However, the therapist encourages the development of positive feelings; if the presence of these positive feelings is brought up by the patient, the therapist accepts them without attempting to have the patient understand anything about them. The patient's positive feelings about the therapist, even if moderately unrealistic, are useful for maintaining the therapeutic alliance and potentially useful identification with the therapist. The therapeutic alliance is discussed further in the next section, in Chapter 2, "Objectives and Mode of Action," and in Chapter 6, "The Therapeutic Relationship." Examples of how transference might be addressed in supportive and expressive psychotherapy follow:

> Patient 1: You always have such a clear way of thinking about things. I'm all over the place, and you always know what the problem is and what to do about it.
>
> Therapist 1: Thanks. It's easier when you hear about it than when you're in the midst of it. (***Supportive psychotherapy***)

> Patient 2: Getting here seems to be more difficult. Things always come up at the last minute. I apologize for being late.
>
> Therapist 2: We could try to change your appointment time if that would help, but I wonder if your finding it more difficult now is because you are having some doubts about continuing. (***Expressive psychotherapy***)

If negative feelings about the therapist or the therapy are evident, or even suspected, they must be discussed, because negative feelings may lead to disruption of treatment. Expressive psychotherapy and supportive psychotherapy approach negative feelings differently. In expressive psychotherapy, the patient's reaction to events in his or her current life may be discussed as possible (unconscious) expressions of the patient's feelings about the therapist:

> Patient: I was on the phone with customer service for half an hour. This really drives me up the wall. It was worse than ever. Those people are incompetent.
>
> Therapist: Last week you were complaining because I hadn't come up with a quick answer for all your problems. Maybe you were especially angry with customer service and saw them as incompetent because you were thinking I was incompetent and you were angry with me.

In supportive psychotherapy, however, events in the therapy may be offered as illustrations or models for everyday life:

> Patient: This really drives me up the wall. It was worse than ever. Those people are incompetent.
>
> Therapist: Last week you were complaining because I hadn't come up with a quick answer for all your problems. You were polite, and we were able to discuss it, and you didn't seem to be "up the wall." Maybe you could be as reasonable and controlled at work as you are here with me.

## Therapeutic Alliance

Competing claims of the many approaches to psychotherapy have given rise to extensive research aimed at discovering just what is the active ingredient in psychotherapy. When it was found that all therapies seem to be effective, one of the research questions asked was "What do all therapies have in common?" That question appears to have been answered. The common element is the *therapeutic alliance* (de Jonghe et al. 1992). If there is a good alliance between patient and therapist, therapy is helpful. If there is not a good alliance, little is accomplished. Therefore, the therapist who is doing supportive and supportive-expressive psychotherapy makes deliberate efforts to encourage a good relationship and avoids actions that are inimical to a good relationship.

Misch (2000) wrote that the therapist should "be a good parent"; this author observed that in one or more psychological domains, the patient is operating ineffectively, so in these domains, the therapist assumes a parental role. Parental behaviors include comforting, soothing, encouraging, nurturing, containment, limit setting, and confronting self-destructive behaviors, all the while encouraging growth and self-sufficiency.

## Self-Esteem

One person helps the self-esteem of another person by conveying acceptance, approval, interest, respect, or admiration. The person whose daily life and relationships lack or are deficient in these qualities may respond to any indication of their presence. The patient who cannot form relationships with others, is avoided by others, or perceives (perhaps correctly) that people look at him or her disapprovingly finds in the therapist a person who is accepting and interested. The therapist's acceptance and trust are unspoken. The therapist communicates his or her interest in the patient by making it evident that he or she remembers their conversations, remembers what the patient has said, and is aware of the patient's likes, dislikes, and attitudes. Acceptance is communicated by avoidance of arguing, denigrating, and criticizing—verbal interactions common to most relationships and, unfortunately, many contacts between patients and health care providers:

> Therapist 1: It doesn't make any sense to get an MRI [magnetic resonance image] just because you forget people's names. *(Argument)*
> Therapist 2: What are you trying to say? *(Denigration)*
> Therapist 3: Didn't they tell you to take it every day? *(Criticism)*

Here are the responses in more congenial language:

Therapist 1: Forgetting names is usually the first defect in memory that normal people experience. If that is the only problem, it's not caused by the sort of thing that shows up on an MRI.
Therapist 2: I don't understand.
Therapist 3: A lot of the effect is lost if you don't take it every day. If the dose is too large, we should discuss it. A smaller dose might be the answer.

Our efforts to boost or avoid lowering the patient's self-esteem require that we avoid language that is overpowering (directly or by implication) and that we avoid behavior that may make the patient feel diminished or helpless—behavior such as pomposity, overelaborate speech, or ostentatiousness. Here are some overpowering statements:

Therapist 1: I'm trying to get you to understand…
Therapist 2: I'm going to medicate you.
Therapist 3: It's your imagination.

And here are better ways to express these ideas:

Therapist 1: I hope I'm being clear.
Therapist 2: Let's talk about medication.
Therapist 3: When you hear something that people around you don't hear, it's not imagination; it's an event in your brain that's not triggered by something in the environment.

Questions that begin with the words *why* or *why didn't you* are often experienced as attacks and should be avoided (Pinsker 1997). In the course of growing up, most people learn that the question "Why did you do it?" is not so much a search for information as a rebuke for having done the particular action. Similarly, "Why didn't you do it?" means "You should have done it." Attack is inimical to self-esteem. Alternatives to "Why?" can be created:

Therapist 1: Can you explain how it was that you did it that way?
Therapist 2: When you dropped out of school, what was the reason?
Therapist 3: Was there something about your behavior that made them think it was necessary to call the police?

Attacking questions are accepted as a matter of course in most relationships, and they are certainly customary in conventional medical practice, so reasonable use of them is not going to destroy the therapy. The goal is to conduct therapy with finesse, thus enhancing prospects for success and for the therapist's satisfaction. In the same vein, when possible, it is better practice to ask questions in a way that elicits a positive response rather than a negative response. For example, it is better to ask an obese person, "Do you find it difficult to exercise?" than to ask "Do you exercise?" It is better to ask a general question, when possible, than a narrow question. For example, "What are you serving for dessert?" is a better question than "Are you serving cake?" The therapist should not be a person to whom the patient must too often answer "No."

The doctor–patient relationship involves a person who has the power to give help and a person who needs help. It is up to the doctor to give this help in a skillful manner that minimizes the inherent inequality of the transaction. The therapist should always respect the patient's individuality and address him or her as an adult. Even severely impaired or disturbed individuals are concerned about their dignity. Respect is good for self-esteem and good for the therapeutic alliance. Even educated, sophisticated patients put up with vague, dismissive explanations by their physicians. They sense that this strategy is more practical than challenging the authority to do better. Below are examples of such dismissive explanations:

Patient 1: I think this medication is making me sleepy.
Physician 1: It hasn't been a problem for most people. How's your appetite?

Patient 2: I don't feel any better.
Physician 2: Well, you look better.

If Physician 2's response is coupled with an explanation that depressed people look better before they feel better, the response is fine. As an abrupt response, it is dismissive and argumentative.

In addition to the self-esteem–building elements of the therapeutic alliance, self-esteem is addressed with specific interventions, which are discussed in Chapter 3, "Interventions (What to Say)."

## Conclusion

Supportive psychotherapy developed out of the practice of psychodynamic psychotherapy. It relies on direct measures to support the patient's defenses, to allay anxiety, and to enhance the patient's adaptive skills. The relationship between patient and therapist—the therapeutic alliance—is recognized as a highly potent element of the treatment, but the alliance becomes a subject for discussion only when problems in the relationship threaten to disrupt treatment.

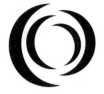

2

# Objectives and Mode of Action

**S**ince Dewald's (1964) exposition of the distinctions between supportive and expressive psychotherapy, there has been universal agreement that although the supportive and expressive ends of the continuum of therapies can be readily contrasted, treatment invariably involves both supportive and expressive elements. Consequently, real-world psychotherapy is supportive-expressive or expressive-supportive, depending on which approach is dominant. The balance could be measured by taping the session and categorizing the therapist's statements (referred to as *interventions* in psychotherapy literature) as either supportive or expressive in intent, but this research strategy offers nothing to the beginning clinician, who must decide from moment to moment what to say next. When summarizing the findings of a detailed study lasting many years and involving 42 patients treated at the Menninger Clinic, Wallerstein (1986) observed that the interface between supportive and expressive psychotherapy could not always be clearly discerned. However, the therapists in this study were experienced psychoanalysts, likely to respond quickly, almost automatically, to the patient's needs. Novice psychotherapists, for whom this book is written, often find themselves using, in a more or less haphazard fashion, all the techniques they have learned—wasting time and reducing the prospects of patient benefit. Responding to everything the patient says is a supportive contaminant when the therapy is psychoanalysis; failure to respond is an analytic contaminant when the treatment is supportive therapy.

The therapist's basic stance is what matters. When the stance is expressive, the therapist follows the dictum "Be as expressive as you can be, and as supportive as you have to be" (Wallerstein 1989, p. 688). When the stance is supportive, the therapist follows Wachtel's (1993) advice: "Be as supportive as you can be so that you can be as expressive as you will need to be" (p. 155).

## Rationale for Conversational Style

The conversational style of supportive psychotherapy defines the procedure as an interaction, not primarily a lesson, not primarily an exploration of mental content, and not an interrogation. Medical students learn to take histories by interrogation—that is, by asking a series of questions. Patients put up with this approach, but such interrogation does not ordinarily make them feel better. Conversational style is quite different from free association, the "say whatever comes to mind" technique of psychoanalysis, in which the immediate objective is to understand the patient's mental life. Use of conversational style does not mean that the therapist jumps in every time the patient stops. Waiting to hear what comes next is as useful in supportive as in expressive therapy. But when the stance is supportive, the therapist will not wait long. Faced with a long pause, the supportive therapist thinks, "Is there any reason why I shouldn't speak?" The expressive therapist, on the other hand, thinks, "Is there an indication for me to speak?"

The therapist's activity reveals much about him or her, and in this way, transference distortion is minimized. The therapist's responsiveness is a form of giving to the patient. The analytic situation is inherently supportive because of the therapist's interest and acceptance. But in supportive psychotherapy, interest and acceptance are not enough. By being responsive, the therapist gives something to the patient. Except for narcissistic individuals, who seem to receive satisfaction from having an audience, people want to be given something in exchange for what they give. This giving, by an intelligent, interested person, is gratifying and reassuring.

The positive relationship, with the therapist conveying that his or her objective is to guide the patient toward improvement, is a direct attack on hopelessness. Interpersonal conflicts, uncertainties about what to do, and anxious feelings are all problems to be solved by developing more effective coping mechanisms. When negative feelings are recognized and discussed, the patient may experience the therapist as being comfortable with hostile feelings, and a source of anxiety is thus removed (Dewald 1994). Many patients treated with supportive psychotherapy have chronic disorders, unsatisfactory living conditions, and little hope of major change. The therapist is a figure of stability, a contact with the outside world, perhaps a representative of the broader world.

The supportive stance supports or ignores defenses when they serve their unconscious purpose—protection of the individual from anxiety or other unpleasant affects. But it is a rare patient whose treatment is entirely supportive. The therapist can support a defense, question a defense, but cannot accept and challenge the same defense simultaneously. We cannot be silent and responsive in the same moment. We cannot simultaneously examine positive feelings and not examine them. We can, however, discuss childhood origins of a problem and also discuss cognitive assumptions that stem from that problem, as well as behavioral strategies for overcoming the problem. Why are childhood origins discussed in a treatment approach that does not attach prime importance to unraveling these origins? Because such discussion is often satisfying to the patient, and because the creation of a biography is a task that patient and therapist work on together, with the patient reaping the benefits of sharing. The biography gives a feeling of certainty. At the same time, the therapist must keep in mind one of the major objectives of supportive psychotherapy or the supportive stance: improvement in the tactics of dealing with the problems of daily life (i.e., improvement of adaptive skills). When treating a severely impaired patient, the therapist may make specific recommendations about what the patient should do (i.e., the therapist may give advice). With most patients, advice is developed out of collaborative discussion about better ways to do things, accompanied by rehearsal of potential problems (anticipatory guidance). The task in expressive psychotherapy, on the other hand, is to understand underlying patterns, with a focus on defenses, so that the patient will develop new and more effective behavior and relationships on his or her own.

## Integration of Supportive and Expressive Elements

The traditional approach to teaching psychotherapy has been to teach expressive theory and practice, leaving the student to figure out what to do in all nonexpressive circumstances. Today the teaching of supportive psychotherapy is added, but the student is still left to decide what to say. As stated earlier in the chapter, the therapist is advised: "Be as supportive as you can be so that you can be as expressive as you will need to be" (Wachtel 1993, p. 155). When does the therapist need to be expressive? Whenever the basic supportive techniques are not enough to accomplish the patient's goals, and whenever it appears that the patient's life can be improved by use of expressive techniques. Expressive measures can be used without altering the supportive stance. Winston and Winston (2002) summarized the matter: "Psychotherapy in general…must be designed to meet the needs of each patient by integrating different psychotherapeutic approaches. These approaches are derived from psychoanalytic, cognitive-behavioral, and interpersonal traditions" (p. 24). We add that the integration includes balancing supportive and expressive elements within a psychodynamic framework.

While the therapist maintains the supportive stance in terms of the therapist–patient relationship, it is permissible and desirable to explore the meaning of the patient's actions and thoughts. Whether a statement that appears to reflect a defensive position is supported, ignored, or questioned depends on the current situation, including the context of the patient–therapist conversation (i.e., does the therapist interrupt the patient to raise a question, or does the therapist go along with the patient's flow, making supportive or accepting comments?). Following are examples of different therapist responses:

Patient: I hated being in the hospital. Every day someone would be acting up and they'd jump on him with a needle. I was glad I wasn't that bad off.

Therapist 1: Maybe you were afraid on some level that it could happen to you. A lot of people equate mental illness with being out of control, so if they find themselves in hospital with mental illness, they are afraid they may be in danger of being out of control. *(Proposal of an explanation for the defense, using the technique of "normalization" to lessen the impact)*

Therapist 2: Yeah. *(Acceptance of the defense without comment)*

Therapist 3: Yes. Your condition was quite different. Severe depression is one thing; a psychotic episode is another. That [a psychotic episode] wouldn't happen to you. *(Encouragement of the defense)*

## Misuse of Therapeutic Tactics

Psychotherapy is a difficult skill. It takes years for most therapists to become able to hear what the patient is saying and to monitor their own words and thoughts. Whereas conducting therapy as a series of questions does not lead to meaningful interaction, the beginning therapist who has overcome the habit of asking follow-up questions is at risk of falling into unproductive agreeableness, always responding to what the patient has just said. For example, the therapist asks a question, the patient gives a partial answer and moves on to another topic, the therapist asks a question about that topic, and the process is repeated—with the therapist never having the opportunity to deal substantially with an issue. Thus beginning therapists are often easily put off: if the patient's answer is not adequate, the therapist asks another question instead of pursuing an answer to the initial question. In short, it is not good form to ask too many questions—but if a question is asked, the issue should not be abandoned without an attempt to get an answer. Here are some examples of different therapeutic tactics:

> Therapist 1: Do you have any thoughts about any issues or events that may have led up to your depression last year? *(Question is worded to avoid use of attacking words* why *or* what.)
>
> Patient: Nothing. It just happened. It came out of the blue.
>
> Therapist 1: Have you ever felt suicidal? *(If the therapist was curious about what led up to the depression, he or she should have attempted to persist with that topic before shifting to a new topic, even though the new topic is relevant.)*
>
> Therapist 2: Well, what was happening in your life in the month or so before the depression began? *(Question does not call on the patient to make cause-and-effect connections.)*
>
> Patient: Nothing special. I went to work. I came home. My husband was working. The kids were in school. *(Uninformative)*
>
> Therapist 2: Let's take these things one at a time. What about work? What were you doing? What about co-workers? Any problems? Did anyone you care about leave? Was your assignment changed? Your supervisor? Any advancement? *(By offering multiple choices, the therapist teaches about topics that might be important.)*
>
> Patient: Not really. Everything was routine. *(Uninformative)*
>
> Therapist 2: OK. Tell me about your husband and children at that time. What was going on? We are looking for things that might have been disturbing but that you might have brushed aside at the time without paying much attention. *(Prodding question is asked in a supportive way.)*

Seeking more complete information about what the patient is saying is a demonstration of interest and attention and is therefore a supportive act, provided the pursuit of additional information does not take on the quality of attack. The key to obtaining complete information is often the wonderful phrase "Give me an example":

> Patient 1: If I get mad at work, I just don't go back.
>
> Therapist 1: Give me an example. Describe the last job you left that way. What was the incident that got to you?
>
> Patient 1: It was nothing. I was working a counter. The customers were arguing with me.
>
> Therapist 1: Exactly what was said? What did the customer say and what did you say?

Patient 2: I have to do everything. My husband is helpless in the house. I come home from work and I have to get dinner, even though he's been home.
Therapist 2: What do you mean, "helpless"? Does he do any tasks at all?

Patient 3: No, I never get angry. I can't remember ever losing my temper.
Therapist 3: Can you describe some instance in which something displeased you a little?

The interpersonal and emotional experiences of early life play important roles in the development of the individual and the development of problems. Examination of these matters is interesting and often useful. It may be demonstrated that responses that were appropriate in the past have been perpetuated even though they are no longer appropriate. The creation of a meaningful autobiography is in itself useful, because what may have appeared to be random events become connected into a meaningful story. Owning a meaningful personal story gives a feeling of mastery. The problem for the beginning therapist, however, is that some patients talk endlessly about their terrible childhoods, emphasizing how they suffered at the hands of others. The inexperienced therapist may allow such talk to go on at length, hopeful that some good will result, with a patient who is avoiding any discussion about changing adaptive patterns or changing his or her manner of relating to people. Ventilation is a legitimate supportive tactic, one that is useful when the patient has been unable to put a painful experience into words (perhaps because he or she has been afraid to or because no one has been there to listen and understand). Recounting the same story may be adaptive when the patient's goal is merely relapse prevention and the therapist's objective is preservation of the status quo; however, such recounting is maladaptive when the goal is to improve life.

Becoming aware of previously unrecognized feelings is extremely important. Once this awareness has been achieved, the general task is to incorporate the awareness into the fabric of memories and life. At one time, many patients' symptoms were related to unacceptable sexual feelings, but now, such connections are much less commonly made. Today, unrecognized anger is a frequently seen problem. Other often hidden feelings include guilt, hopelessness, and grief that was not experienced at the time of an important loss. It is now well established that "getting the anger out" is not usually helpful and is often counterproductive. Some individuals are scarcely aware of any feelings at all (the term *alexithymia* has been used to describe this condition). For such persons, an important objective is to recognize, acknowledge, identify, and label emotions (Misch 2000).

The beginning therapist often asks "How did it feel?" or "How does it feel?" in response to almost anything the patient says, and then the therapist goes on to something else. Feelings connected to events in the past should be explored if the therapist and patient are working on the problem of unrecognized feelings or are examining coping strategies, or if the therapist is seeking opportunities to expand his or her empathic understanding. Often, with respect to current feelings, the discussion topic must be "What is going to be done about it?" The question "What did you think?" is as useful as "What did you feel?" because it pertains to thought process, reality testing, or adaptive skills. In short, the person who knows only thoughts and does not know feelings needs to feel more, and the person who feels too much needs to think and evaluate more. Usually, however, therapeutic dialogue involves both feelings and thoughts. Jumping to adaptive solutions without understanding the patient's emotional response is as wrong as ignoring adaptive strategies.

## Mode of Action

The question of what is happening when psychotherapy is effective has been examined at length. Although overlapping, the purely supportive element and the expressive element must be addressed separately.

Attempts to achieve the supportive psychotherapy objectives of improved ego function and adaptive skills involve teaching, encouragement, exhortation, modeling, and anticipatory guidance. People in general, not only patients, respond to teaching and instruction if they want to learn, if they want to improve their lot, and if they trust the teacher. They may cooperate with the teacher to please him or her. Such cooperation has been described in psychoanalytic writing as a "transference cure." The Menninger psychotherapy research project found that changes that appeared to come about for this reason proved stable and durable (Wallerstein 1986).

Alexander and French (1946) introduced the term *corrective emotional experience*. A patient's transference may cause him or her to unconsciously perceive the therapist as having attributes associated with unpleasant interactions in the past. However, the therapist does not respond like the figure from the past, and in time, the old feelings become muted and the patient no longer needs to replay new relationships according to the old emotional script. This result, according to the theory, is accomplished without explicit analysis. Corrective emotional experiences may occur at any point of the continuum of psychopathology or the continuum of psychotherapies.

The concept of *change* occurs throughout the literature on psychotherapy. At one end of the continuum, *change* means lasting personality change. At the other end, sought-for changes may concern specific behaviors, such as sitting in front of the television all day, skipping medications, spending money foolishly, remaining in a bad environment, or failing to control children. If simple advice is all it takes to get the patient to change his or her habitual behavior, it is not necessary to do more. Often, however, there are obstacles in the way of change that the patient does not verbalize. If the therapist is to give useful advice, he or she must be familiar with the psychological and emotional problems that may be operating.

> Therapist 1: The last time you were here, we talked about the support group, and you said you were going to talk to the social worker about it. I wonder what happened that you didn't. *("What happened?" is not as attacking as "Why?")*
> Patient 1: I don't know. I had trouble with my car. I had to go to the dentist.
> Therapist 1: I know a lot of people have trouble doing too many things in one week. Overscheduling is also an easy habit to get into, and not a good one. *(Normalizing, exhorting, judgmental)*
>
> Therapist 2: People who have not been able to do much for a long time— it can happen with illness—become fearful of doing new things. They think they will do something wrong or that they won't know how to fit in. Does that make any sense? *(Teaching; confronting, i.e., bringing to the patient's attention feelings or thoughts outside his or her awareness)*
> Patient 1: I get very nervous when I meet new people.
> Therapist 2: So we have to find a way to deal with the nervousness that will make it possible for you to have the interview with the social worker. After that, you can think about whether the group might be useful for you. *(Scolding replaced by acceptance; moving toward constructive efforts)*

This vignette illustrates how even in work with the most impaired individuals, the therapist must explore feelings and ideas of which the patient is not aware. This approach is an expressive element. If responsibility for the patient is to go beyond simplest take-it-or-leave-it advice, beyond criticizing the patient for being noncompliant, the therapy must be psychodynamically oriented supportive psychotherapy or expressive-supportive psychotherapy (Luborsky 1984).

## Psychodynamics for the Absolute Beginner

Many physicians begin psychiatric training without having had exposure to psychodynamics or any form of psychotherapy. Some trainees are from countries where psychodynamic thinking has not been widely disseminated. These physicians may not know what to talk about with the patient after completing the history, and they may believe that in some way, if the patient talks about his or her past and feelings, he or she will do well. Therefore, for the absolute beginner (and no one else), we offer a few words about psychodynamics.

Psychodynamics is the interaction between conscious and unconscious elements of mental life and is an explanation of the meaning of behavior. One of the tasks of psychotherapy is to make order out of symptoms and dysfunctions. To accomplish this order, the patient and therapist join in developing a history in which these symptoms and dysfunctions make sense. Cause-and-effect connections are established, although different schools of psychodynamic thinking may derive different explanations at times. However, the process of making a comprehensible story may be what matters most. Here are a few illustrations of psychodynamic formulations:

- A man who is ordinarily self-sufficient and cheerful becomes demanding and uncooperative when hospitalized after a heart attack, although he has been reassured that the prognosis is good. A psychodynamic hypothesis might be that the passive, somewhat helpless role of hospital patient is anxiety provoking, and the patient is attempting to compensate by assuming an overbearing attitude. Because he is not aware that the enforced passivity is behind his unusual behavior, we call his behavior unconscious.
- After being criticized by his parents for watching television all night, a schizophrenic patient stops taking his antipsychotic medication. According to his chart, patient education has been provided, and the patient has verbalized understanding. The patient has become angry with his parents. He is not aware that "forgetting" to take his medication is psychologically motivated defiance.
- Home for Thanksgiving during his first year of college, a healthy teenager provokes a big argument the day before he leaves, with the consequence that when he leaves, he is angry. He is not aware that part of him (not all) would like to stay home (and be dependent). By going away angry, he is protected from the sadness that is part of the picture.
- A patient comes regularly for clinic visits, each time giving a detailed account of how other people abuse her. After many attempts to get the patient to examine her role in causing or maintaining at least some of her troubles, the therapist suggests that therapy is unproductive and should be discontinued because it will be seen as poor utilization of resources. A psychodynamic hypothesis might be that because repeating

familiar patterns is an anxiety-reducing element of human behavior, the patient may be setting up a situation in which she will be rejected, thus confirming her expectations about relationships with people.

An important assumption of psychodynamically oriented therapies is that unrecognized emotions are often responsible for current unpleasant feelings or maladaptive behavior and that becoming aware of these emotions may provide relief. More often, the discovery of an unrecognized emotion must be followed by conscious decisions about more effective methods of coping—the adaptive skills focus of supportive psychotherapy. As stated previously, beginners often ask "How did you feel?" without having a specific intent or a plan about what to do with the answer. The question is pertinent when it initiates discussion of 1) how the patient dealt with the feeling; or 2) if there was no feeling, discussion of the possibility that this lack is of itself an important finding:

> Patient: I asked the guy next door to go to the mall with me, but he said he didn't have time. He doesn't have any more to do than I do.
> Therapist: How did you feel about that?
> Patient: It's all right. He doesn't have to. *(Evasive, denying emotional response)*
> Therapist: You're right. He doesn't have to. That's a correct analysis. *(Praise)* But you're offering an analysis when I asked about your feelings. *(Confrontation; implied question)*
> Patient: I didn't feel anything.
> Therapist: You describe a situation in which most people would feel disappointment or anger—that [disappointment or anger] won't control the other person, but it's important to know what your feelings are because when you don't, you can't make good decisions about things that affect you. *(Teaching, normalizing)*

Another tenet of psychodynamically oriented therapy is that people often follow patterns of behavior that were appropriate when established but that have become maladaptive. For example, during adolescence, when it is important to reduce emotional dependency on parents, many people assume a belligerent or defiant style. This attitude may be appropriate at age 16 but may be a continual source of trouble at age 26, 46, or 66. Some people—once they see that they are clinging to a pattern of behavior that is familiar, understandable, but no longer useful—are able, with determined effort, to change their habitual responses. Cognitive-behavioral therapy focuses on the assumptions associated with patterns and provides tactics for overcoming these assumptions. Although cognitive and psychodynamic approaches are usually taught separately, tactics of both approaches are integrated in everyday treatment.

Psychodynamic explanations tell us about the interplay of factors in current life; they do not explain the origins of the forces, emotions, or assumptions that affect behavior. *Psychogenetics* is the search for these origins. If we say that a man seeking to have sexual relationships with as many women as possible has "a Don Juan syndrome," we are making a diagnosis (a syndrome diagnosis, not a DSM diagnosis). If we say that he acts this way to compensate for insecurity about his masculinity, we are making a psychodynamic hypothesis. If we say that he is insecure because he was afraid of his overbearing father, we are proposing a psychogenetic hypothesis.

Consider another situation: A man in his late 30s is readily able to form relationships but always ends them by discovering faults in his partner and shifting from loving behavior to quarreling. A psychodynamic possibility is that he is unconsciously fearful of closeness or intimacy. The search for patterns that may explain symptoms or maladaptive behavior is the expressive component of supportive-expressive psychotherapy. As soon as we get past the history-eliciting phase of treatment, we are concerned first about feelings and assumptions that are present but unexpressed, then about feelings and assumptions that are lightly concealed, and only later about feelings and assumptions that have been truly hidden. A long-familiar analogy is that psychotherapy is like peeling an onion.

Films and plays of the 1950s often show a patient in psychotherapy or psychoanalysis discovering an early traumatic experience and immediately recovering. In real life once the discoveries are made, usually the patient must make great efforts to change his or her ways of thinking and responding. The importance of explaining origins is not as great as once thought, but an explanation of origins still has its uses. Although becoming physically abusive is not an invariable result of previous physical abuse, people who were beaten when they were children are more likely to be physically abusive adults than are people who did not have this unfortunate experience. The methods of cognitive-behavioral therapy, many of which have been incorporated into supportive psychotherapy, may be the principal approach once the patient sees that the behavior causing him or her distress is the outcome of a plausible story.

Education and instruction are potent agents for bringing about change in people's lives. Advice and instruction are most likely to be followed when given by a person one trusts and respects. The skillful therapist and the skillful teacher give the instruction that is needed, at the time when it can be absorbed and used. The patient's mother may have said, "Clean your room." The psychotherapist teaches, "It's not good for your self-esteem to be surrounded by evidence that you can't keep order in your life." Sometimes, this approach is all it takes to bring about change. Possible causes of maladaptive behavior need be sought only when advice doesn't work. It is remarkable how often, when a patient mentions a former therapist, he or she tells us what that therapist told him or her to do.

## Conclusion

Supportive psychotherapy is conducted in conversational style, involving examination of the patient's current and past experiences, responses, and feelings. Although the initial focus is on self-esteem, ego function, and adaptive skills, the therapeutic alliance may be the most important element of the therapy. The therapist seeks to expand the patient's self-mastery by helping him or her to become aware of thoughts and feelings outside awareness and to provide specific suggestions for more adaptive living.

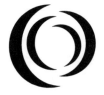

# 3

# Interventions
# (What to Say)

**W**hen we support someone, we use measures designed to keep him or her from falling, from being unable to function. We want the person to feel better and function better. The purely supportive techniques of praise, reassurance, and encouragement—significant components of supportive-expressive therapy—are directed primarily at self-esteem concerns. By his or her attitude, the therapist conveys acceptance, respect, and interest. At the same time, in countless ways, the therapist models adaptive, reasonable, organized behavior and thinking.

## Praise

It is good supportive technique to express praise abundantly. Praise can be sprinkled into conversation as salt from a saltshaker. Praise may be reinforcement of accomplishments or of more adaptive behaviors, provided that the patient is likely to agree that praise is deserved. Here are some illustrations:

> Therapist 1: Telling your mother that you knew you had been nasty was a good step. Do you agree?
> Therapist 2: You're able to make this very clear.
> Therapist 3: It's good that you can be so considerate of other people.
> *(Note, however, that in some contexts, being too considerate may be seen*

*as a symptom, and a statement that the patient is too considerate*
*might serve as a confrontation.)*

False praise or praise that is meaningless to the patient is worse than saying nothing. Falsity and deception are incompatible with any good relationship.

Patient: I was always afraid of my mother.
Therapist: What were you afraid of?
Patient: She came in this morning and said, "Why are you still in bed?"
  She doesn't respect me. They argue a lot. I was 15 before I realized
  that she was crazy.
Therapist 1: You explained that well. (*A supportive comment, but in this*
  *instance, a lie. The patient has mixed past and present and has*
  *mixed his mother's attitude toward him and her relationship with*
  *her husband. Thought-disordered responses can be "decoded," but*
  *the patient cannot be said to have explained his situation well.*)
Therapist 2: It's hard for you to describe these things. You're making a big
  effort. (*Accurate and useful*)

When the therapist expresses praise for something that the patient cannot feel good about, the therapist's words will be ineffective and may even have a negative effect.

Patient (a graduate student before he became disabled): I really have been
  feeling bad. I don't do anything. I manage to eat, but most of the
  time I'm a blob.
Therapist: Did you do anything last week besides sit around at home?
  (*The therapist is not content with the global self-description and*
  *seeks specifics.*)
Patient: Well, I went to a movie...
Therapist: That's great!!!
Patient: Yeah.
(*The therapist didn't understand that for this patient, the fact that he was*
  *able to do nothing better than go to one movie represents failure.*)

An important strategy for preventing communication-failure is to seek feedback.

Patient: Well, I went to a movie...
Therapist: That's great! What do you think? Weren't you pleased with
  yourself? (*Seeking feedback*)
Patient: Not really. It's nothing. I used to be active all day and all night. If
  the most I can do is go to a stupid movie, I'm in bad shape.
Therapist: But it's good that you got out. It's a change. It's a good step.
  (*Arguing, making the situation worse. The therapist should have*
  *engaged the patient by returning to his bad feelings.*)

Find opportunities to respond with honest praise. How often should the therapist praise? When praise is given too often, it may seem contrived or insincere. The healthier the patient (the further to the right on the psychopathology scale), the less praise is called for. At the far right on the psychopathology scale, praise should be limited to situations in which it is the socially expected response (e.g., congratulations for accomplishment). It may be useful to compliment a patient for persisting with an anxiety-provoking topic in the therapy. The easiest praise comes from the therapist's approval of what the patient is doing. Such praise, however, is opinion or judgment. The best praise is reinforcement of the patient's steps toward achieving previously stated goals.

> Patient: I took my lithium every day last week.
> Therapist 1: Good. (***Judgmental, but appropriately so***)
> Therapist 2: Good. That gives you a good chance to avoid another episode. (***Reinforcing desirable behavior, but still authoritarian***)
> Therapist 3: Good. You said you were going to do this—not skip a single dose—and you did it. (***Reinforcing self-control and discipline***)
> ....What do you think? (***Continuing the conversation by seeking feedback and further engagement***)

A general principle of psychotherapy is to avoid contradicting or arguing, although at times it is difficult to distinguish between arguing, reframing, and giving appropriate attention to adaptive skills.

> Patient: I feel as bad as ever. I don't think the medication is any good.
> Therapist 1: You look a lot better to me. (***A contradiction; often occurs in physician–patient discourse***)
> Therapist 2: People who are recovering from depression usually look better and eat better as the medication begins to work, and they look better and eat better before they feel better. (***Disagreement, but the therapist is conveying expert information that may be useful to the patient***)
> Therapist 3: You have to get up and do things. You can't stay in bed all day waiting to feel better. (***Argumentative, and true only after antidepressants have proved effective***)
> Therapist 4: If you had continued taking the medication as you were supposed to, you wouldn't be in this position. (***Obnoxious***)

## Reassurance

Reassurance is a familiar tactic in general medicine. Like praise, reassurance must be honest. As with praise, the patient must believe that the reassurance is based on an understanding of his or her unique situation. Reassurance that is given before the patient has detailed his or her concerns is likely to be doubted. Further, the psychotherapist or physician, as an expert, must limit reassurance to areas in which he or she has expert knowledge or dependable common information. We can reassure a patient about effects and side effects of a medication, but we cannot reassure a patient about long-term effects of a medication that has just come on the market. We can say, when true, that no side effects have been reported. It is correct to say that most people recover within a few weeks from an acute episode of psychosis and that most people recover from bereavement within a year or so, but it is never correct to say that a treatment is certain to be successful. We can tell a person with schizophrenia that the disease often stops getting worse after some years and later may begin to improve. We can reassure a patient with chronic illness that we will continue to provide care, because our continuing concern may matter more than cure. It is never acceptable to offer reassurance that is simply what the patient (or family) wants to hear. If the patient demands reassurance and this reassurance is outside the expertise of the therapist, the basis for the reassurance should be made explicit.

> Patient: All day long when my son is in school, I'm sure something bad is going to happen.
> Therapist: You see terrible things on the news, but you know the odds are that nothing bad happens to most people most of the time. (***This is not expert knowledge; it is based on knowledge that comes from general education and popular information.***)
> Patient: And I'm having a hard time finding food that isn't genetically modified. It's dangerous. The people in stores don't know, and I get the runaround when I call the 800 numbers.
> Therapist: I know a lot of people are worried about this, but from what I read in the paper, there have been no reports of anything actually happening to anyone. (***All the therapist knows is what he reads in the papers.***)
> ***The therapist's role, in the face of fearfulness about the unknown, is to teach strategies for dealing with the fearfulness, not to reassure it away.***

*Normalizing*, for most people, is a palatable form of reassurance.

> Patient 1: When my grandmother died, I didn't really feel bad. My mother was so upset, but I wasn't. It makes me feel guilty.
> Therapist 1: It's not unusual. Unless there's a very close relationship, children often seem to accept the death of a grandparent as a matter of course. (***Normalizing and possibly absolution***)

> Patient 2: When I came out to my parents, my mother wanted to know what she had done wrong, and my father acted like I was a criminal. I still hate them.

Therapist 2: We know that this happened a lot of the time. When your parents were young and forming their knowledge of the world, the experts said that homosexuality was caused by parents doing something wrong. Also, in those days, homosexuality was classified as a subtype of psychopathic personality. Haven't you come across other gay men who had similar experiences with their parents and who feel the same way about them now as you do about your parents? (*The therapist normalizes the patient's feelings and encourages understanding rather than expression of feeling.*)

Patient 3: I know I shouldn't be in this program. I'll never understand Lacan.

Therapist 3: Neither will I. (*Using oneself as a standard is risky, but here, the therapist assumes she will be seen as a representative educated person and the patient's peer.*)

Adages and maxims are a form of normalizing, as in the following examples:

Therapist 1: You can't make your [adult] children like each other! (*Reassurance given as an authority*)

Therapist 2: I don't know of studies, but we know from newspapers, literature, and the Bible that siblings often don't get along. (*Normalizing reassurance given as an educated person*)

Therapist 3: There's a saying: "You can't make your child eat, sleep, or be happy." I guess we could add "or get along with a brother or sister." (*Normalizing using a maxim*)

Therapist 4: I have never liked my brother either. (*Inappropriate self-disclosure that serves no useful purpose and crosses the boundaries of the professional relationship*)

Reassurance and normalizing must not extend to pathological and non-adaptive behavior, nor to opportunistic, hostile interactions with others. The objectives of supportive psychotherapy are most effectively advanced when reassurance is coupled with enunciation of a principle or a rule:

Patient: Whenever I go anywhere, I have this fear that I'm going to lose control.

Therapist 1: You won't lose control. (*Reassurance as an authority is useful but not as potent as reassurance that reinforces the patient's strengths or adaptive skills.*)

Therapist 2: I don't think you will lose control. You have had this fear for a long time, and you have always been able to maintain good self-control. (*Reassurance based on the patient's history, and reinforcement of adaptive behavior*)

Therapist 3: People with social phobia always fear losing control; however, actually losing control is not part of the condition. (*Reassurance based on a principle*)

# Encouragement

Encouragement too has a major role in general medicine and rehabilitation. Patients with chronic schizophrenia, depression, or a passive-dependent style are often inactive, mentally and physically. The therapist encourages the patient to maintain hygiene, to get exercise, to interact with other people, sometimes to be more independent, and sometimes to accept the care and concern of others. Rehabilitation requires small steps. Many people discount small steps, seeing each step as of no great importance. Therapy with disabled persons calls for ingenuity in identifying tasks and activities that can be conceptualized as small steps.

> Patient 1: I don't see why I should waste time in occupational therapy. I'm not going to get a job painting flowerpots.
>
> Therapist 1: OT isn't intended to be job training for flowerpot painting. The idea is to allow people to have the experience of staying in one place and completing a task—that can be a problem for some; it's about being able to cope with detail, with structure. It's also, for some people, an opportunity to stop thinking about one's psyche or problems. (***Addresses both the "small steps" element and the diversion element***)

> Patient 2: I'm tired of not getting anywhere. My father is willing to pay, and I'm going to start college in the fall.
>
> Therapist 2: Before you take such a big step, I'd suggest taking an adult education course at the high school or community college. It wouldn't be all that you want, but it's a low-risk way to see if you can handle regular attendance, pay attention, turn in assignments, and just feel comfortable with other people. (***Enrolling in a degree program and failing is not effective rehabilitation; it is bad for self-esteem. This intervention might also be categorized as advice.***)

Encouragement is powerful because people want to believe that their efforts will lead to something. Encouragement invokes the world of childhood, where adults do things for the child's benefit. *Exhortation* is a more insistent form of encouragement.

> Patient: I'm eating OK, I sleep well, but I can't get going. My apartment's a mess. And they want me to take one of those "welfare" jobs.
>
> Therapist: A demoralized person is convinced his or her efforts will come to nothing, so the person doesn't try. The only way out of it, once the depression is better, is to force yourself to begin doing things even though you don't feel like it. Living in a mess that reminds you every day that you can't function is bad for your self-esteem, too, so forcing yourself to clean up ought to be helpful.

The discussion of encouragement thus far has dealt with only one of the two meanings of the word *encourage*—that is, "to stimulate, to spur." The other meaning is "to give hope." The following dialogue illustrates the use of encouragement to give a patient hope.

Patient: All I was able to do last week was go to a movie. I must be in bad shape.

Therapist: One of the worst things about depression is that it makes you unable to even imagine things being better. Everything that was ever good is new evidence of how bad you are now. That's the illness. It may be hard to believe, but these medications usually make a difference and the depression lifts. For now, do what you can. Does this make any sense?

## Rationalizing and Reframing

Reframing involves looking at something in a different light or from a different perspective:

Patient: I was so stupid. I got a parking ticket, and I could have been back before the meter ran out. I wasn't paying attention.

Therapist: Yeah. That's tough. If you figure it's bound to happen occasionally, you can think of a couple of parking tickets a year as a routine cost of having a car. (**Rationalization. The patient also benefits *from discovering that the therapist, who represents the adult world, does not think she is stupid.***)

The challenge in using rationalizing and reframing is to avoid sounding fatuous and to avoid what may appear to be argument or contradiction. Reframing should provide a welcome new way of looking at things:

Patient: My son keeps his room such a mess. It's impossible. He knows it drives me up the wall. My husband says, "Don't go in his room," but I can't just ignore it.

Therapist: You know, I suppose that a lot of 15-year-old boys are like that. I wonder why you can't act on what you know. (**Normalizing and *trying to select a topic in which the patient, not another person, is the subject***)

Patient: I think he does it to spite me. It wouldn't take much for him to keep it neat. (**Ignoring the therapist's words**)

Therapist: If we think of your son's keeping his room messy as a rebellion against you, it can be seen as a fairly safe way of doing something on his own without getting in trouble, and we can see that you have given him enough sense of security that he can begin to act on his own. This may be an indication that you've done things right. (**Reframing**)

# Important Topics for Therapeutic Conversation

The beginning therapist knows how to take a history and how to make a clinical diagnosis, knows that events of the past bear on the present, but may not know what to talk about with a new patient. We always start with what the patient wants to talk about, but then the therapist must decide whether it will be useful to dwell on that topic or move on to others that experience teaches are often fruitful or important. When the patient has recently been hospitalized, medications are a priority topic. The first concern is whether he or she is experiencing any unwanted or uncomfortable effects. When patients don't take medication as prescribed, physicians often express their frustration by criticizing the patient for noncompliance. Paying attention to untoward effects helps to transform the matter from adversarial to collaborative. Psychological issues may also play a part, such as not wanting to feel overpowered and not wanting to accept the existence of illness.

Details of daily life should be discussed with the nonfunctioning individual, and the therapist should watch for opportunities for improving adaptive skills. We want to know how the patient understands his or her condition and what feelings are related to it. A person who has a chronic disabling condition, unless effectively a denier, ought to have the opportunity to talk about the condition. Often the person has fears about the future that are not expressed. Depression accompanies many conditions. Depression may be a response to discovering that one faces a life of disability or a response to looking back over lost years and family tension.

The therapist should know about the people in the patient's life. Higher-functioning patients are likely to have important relationships, to think about their interactions, and to bring up these interactions for discussion. Lower-functioning patients (and some aged individuals) may lead lives almost devoid of relationships and may talk at length about their symptoms or may talk abstractly about their mental problems. They may talk extensively about intrafamily events of childhood, never saying anything about current life. The therapist should know about family, friends, acquaintances, co-workers, and, in the case of isolated patients, persons with whom the patient has even brief contact, such as case workers, probation officers, receptionists, guards, and waiters and waitresses. Questions and statements therapists might use to obtain information about patient contacts are presented here:

Therapist 1: Did you have contact with anyone in the last few days?
Patient 1: My sister-in-law called.
Therapist 1: Tell me about her.

Patient 1: She's gross.
Therapist 1: Can you describe her? (***Broader and less demanding question than "Why don't you like her?"***)

Therapist 2: Who are the people in your life now?
Patient 2: No one. The only people I know use drugs.
Therapist 2: Is there someone you talk to most days?

Therapist 3: You say your son will come if you call him. Does that mean he doesn't come if you don't call?
Patient 3: He'll drop what he's doing if we need him, but...to come on a Sunday afternoon? Forget it.

Therapist 4: Tell me about the people who live in the residence.

Therapist 5: Girlfriend? Is this someone you've known for some time?

*Prevention of relapse* is an important supportive psychotherapy objective. If we turn to the substance abuse literature, we find practical lists of topics to discuss (Marlatt and Gordon 1985, pp. 71–104). It takes little imagination to modify these lists slightly to apply them to the needs of the nonaddicted mentally ill:

- Identification of high-risk situations, and anticipatory guidance for dealing with them
- Coping with negative emotional states
- Coping with interpersonal conflict
- Coping with social pressure
- Identifying relapse, and anticipatory guidance for dealing with relapse

## Advice and Teaching

Advice is an important tactic of supportive psychotherapy. The challenge for the therapist is knowing when to move from giving advice to helping patients learn to find their own way or to find their own sources of advice and information. Offering advice to a dependent person can be gratifying but may deprive the patient of the opportunity to grow.

If the patient senses that the therapist is proposing advice that is not clearly a response to the patient's needs (e.g., that reflects the therapist's prejudices or convictions), the alliance will be damaged. In the following dialogue, Therapist 2 offers a more helpful explanation of advice given:

Therapist: You should get regular exercise.
Patient: What for?

Therapist 1: Everyone should. Obesity is a major problem in this country. (***Possibly true, but the statement is presented as a general truth; the patient must infer the relevance of the statement***)

Therapist 2: A number of studies have shown that exercise reduces symptoms of depression. It can reduce the amount of medication needed. If you do it and it doesn't help, you haven't lost much.

Advice is meaningful when the patient sees it as pertinent to his or her needs. If the advice is a good idea but not in step with the patient's perceived needs, it is like a commercial or a sermon: possibly true, but not personal. A patient who hears advice that seems to be boilerplate, or who hears praise that is false, may experience such comments as another instance of being dependent on someone who fails to meet his or her needs.

Advice and teaching are appropriate in areas in which the therapist is professionally expert: mental illness, normal human behavior, interpersonal transactions, and, possibly, participation in hierarchical organizations. Examples of advice given by therapists follow:

Therapist 1: Taking an entry-level job would be a big comedown, but when a person hasn't worked for a long time and doesn't have connections, it's often the only way to get back into the work world. If you later attempt to get back to your old level, the entry-level job provides evidence to a prospective employer that you have returned to the point where you get to work and do a day's work.

Therapist 2: People who are interested in what you do usually don't want all the details. They may be interested to know that you enjoyed a movie, but they may not want to hear the whole story. Try stopping and noticing whether the other person asks a question that would tell you he or she wants to know more.

It is appropriate to give advice about activities of daily living to seriously impaired patients:

Therapist 1: When you get up in the morning, you should get dressed and make your bed. It's important to have a structure and a routine.

Therapist 2: They offer you free credit, but you're better off not getting into debt. (***Mature wisdom***)

Therapist 3: Let's see if we can work out a strategy about what you should do when you are upset, so you don't have to come to the emergency room and say you are suicidal. (***Adaptive skills***)

Therapist 4: I think you should make a plan to begin cleaning up your apartment, because it's bad for your self-esteem to be surrounded by evidence of your inability to function. (***Rationale is explained.***)

Therapist 5: If you don't do something about your apartment, it's possible that someone will make a complaint to the health department. (***Anticipatory guidance that sounds critical***)

Advice about activities of daily living should not be given to persons who are not impaired, even though this advice might make their lives better.

The therapist should not give advice on issues about which the patient can make his or her own decisions. Such advice is a feature of social conversation, not of psychotherapy, as the therapist in the following dialogue recognizes:

> Patient: You know I worry about everything. Do you think it's safe to use my credit card on the Internet? I read that they can steal your identity…
>
> Therapist: Yes, I've read about that. I think the psychotherapy question is not whether I think it's a good idea but how you come to a decision when there are different opinions or when you have competing pressures.

Advice is generally safe when it is based on what the patient has reported; advice based on surmise, although the advice is sought by the patient, is unprofessional:

> Patient: My boyfriend humiliated me in public again yesterday. I screamed at him when we got home, and he said I was too sensitive. I can't take it anymore.
>
> Therapist 1: Tell him that if he does this again, you are leaving. (***Unless the therapist is totally aware of the unconscious forces that have kept the couple together, such advice should be left for friends to give. If the patient leaves and is then unhappy, she may blame the therapist.***)
>
> Therapist 2: If the pattern you've described holds, it's likely that things will be all right for a while and then it will happen again. (***Might be taken as implicit advice***)
>
> Therapist 3: Have you considered couples therapy? (***Possibly good advice, although at times suggesting more therapy or a new therapist is used as a tactic for ending discussion***)

Teaching is more important than advice. Teaching involves principles, which may be based on technical knowledge or the therapist's position as a rational, informed person familiar with the unwritten rule book of life. In supportive psychotherapy literature, the term *lending ego* has been used to convey that the therapist models reasonable, controlled behavior in addition to teaching about it. He or she gives advice about or teaches about the supportive psychotherapy objectives of improving ego function and adaptive skills, as shown in the following examples:

> Therapist 1: You tend to put up with things until you become furious; then, for example, you scream at people. Dealing with a problem before it becomes extreme is usually a better approach.

Therapist 2: Even if you are right, people do not like to be told what to do.

Therapist 3: His name is on the door, not yours.

Therapist 4: People who are demoralized are convinced that their efforts will not succeed, so they don't try. When this happens, it's important to make an effort to get going. It's hard, because when a person is severely depressed, efforts may fail, and this is even worse for self-esteem.

## Anticipatory Guidance

Rehearsal, or anticipatory guidance, is a technique as useful in supportive psychotherapy as in cognitive-behavioral therapy. The objective is to consider in advance what obstacles there might be to a proposed course of action, and then to prepare strategies for dealing with them. With more impaired patients, the guidance must be more concrete:

Therapist: What's your plan?

Patient: I'm going to begin reintegrating into society. (***Nonspecific***)

Therapist: What will be your first step? (***Aware that a nonspecific, vague response is not a plan***)

Patient: Well, maybe I'll go to the senior center. My son's wife said she'd drive me and bring me home.

Therapist: Can you think of any problems that could come up?

Patient: She might have to stay late at work…

Therapist: What could you do if that happened?

Patient: The senior center is near the library. I could wait there, I suppose.

Therapist: Good idea. What else? How do you think you will react to being there?

Patient: I won't know anyone.

Therapist: That's hard for almost anyone. What will you do?

Patient: I suppose I could introduce myself to someone who doesn't look too senile.

Therapist: Yes. And maybe you could ask the director or someone in charge to introduce you to a few people. People running these programs appreciate that it's hard for a newcomer.

Patient: I suppose so.

Therapist: What if you give it a few days and still don't feel good about it?

The dialogue above illustrates a straightforward use of this technique. Anticipatory guidance is particularly important for patients with chronic schizophrenia, because these individuals are especially likely to be apprehensive in new situations, unsure of their ability to grasp social cues, unsure of appropriate responses, fearful of rejection, and unable to maintain a prolonged effort. The substance abuse patient, too, fears rejection and may unwittingly invite it.

Anticipatory guidance can be helpful and supportive in contexts other than rehabilitation:

Patient: I'm seeing my internist next week about this indigestion and weakness.

Therapist: You know, I hope, that you should start with the most distressing symptom and not at the beginning. Are you willing to rehearse what you will say to explain your problem to the doctor?

Patient: OK. . . . I've been feeling generally bad for 3 months, and for about 3 weeks, I've felt nauseated almost every day. It's worse after I eat.

Therapist: Good! And if anyone says, "Do you understand?" and you are not completely sure, say, "Would you go over it again?"

# Reducing and Preventing Anxiety

The supportive psychotherapist intends not only to deal with overt anxiety, a symptom, but to prevent emergence of anxiety. Some of the measures intended to accomplish these objectives have already been discussed, such as reassurance and encouragement. Every effort is made to avoid the interrogative style, which involves asking continuous questions, giving little, and not making the intent of the questions known to the patient—the style of a trial attorney cross-examining a witness or conducting a deposition. To minimize anxiety, the therapist shares his or her agenda with the patient, making clear the reason for questions or topics:

Therapist 1: I want to ask questions that will test your memory and concentration.

Therapist 2: Your relationship with your daughter, you said, was a major worry. Is there anything new there?

Therapist 3: Did you grieve when your father died? Some people have little response, and it's all right, but some don't have any response at the time but have it bottled up.

Note that Therapist 3 gives extra explanation. The use of extra words—even an excessive number of words, as is often done by an evasive individual—adds padding and reduces the impact. The supportive psychotherapist avoids forcing the patient out on a limb, requiring him or her to make a stark response. In the following statements, the two therapists are trying to obtain the same information, but in different ways:

Therapist 1: Do you experience sexual stimulation when you see someone being hurt by another person? (***Blunt***)

Therapist 2: This may seem like an odd question, but it's relevant when someone has had as much physical conflict as you have had. Do you sometimes experience sexual stimulation in connection with someone inflicting pain? In connection with pictures of torture? This could include paintings of martyrs in museums. It's not rare. All those great paintings show that a lot of people have found excuses to portray and look at torture. On the other hand, a person can be involved in a lot of violence and not have this response. (*If the patient says, "No," he is not in conflict with the therapist, because the patient has been given permission to say "No." If the patient says, "Yes," he is in good company.*)

Telling the patient in advance that something might be anxiety producing is an effective tactic for minimizing the occurrence of anxiety in the treatment. This technique is one of several important and useful interventions enunciated by Pine (1984). For example, a therapist might say the following:

> Therapist: I want to return to a topic that we had to leave once because it upset you. I'd like to know more about what happened when your mother remarried and his children moved in.

One can be even more protective by asking the patient to give permission to go on with an anxiety-provoking topic:

> Therapist [*continuing*]: Do you think you can handle it?

## Naming the Problem

The patient's sense of control may be enhanced, and thus anxiety minimized, by naming problems. The need for control is one reason why human beings find pleasure in counting and classifying. In the following dialogue, the therapist names the patient's problem:

> Patient: I'm so stupid. I had all those people for dinner, and I didn't allow enough time for the rice to cook, and I thought I was smart to make salads early but then there wasn't enough room in the refrigerator, and I didn't think to ask everyone if they ate meat. What kind of example am I for my daughter? How can I talk about taking courses if I can't get the laundry done?
>
> Therapist: Sounds like this is just evidence of your organization problem. We have talked about it, and you have made progress. Let's talk about some specific things you might have done differently. (*The objective of "de-catastrophizing" is approached by reducing what appears to be a multitude of problems to a single problem with a name.*)

Naming the problem is also meeting the familiar medical responsibility of explaining the diagnosis, prognosis, and proposed treatment:

> Patient: My mother says I shouldn't lie down so much, but it feels better when I do. I read the ads every week, but the jobs don't pay enough, and there's no future. I don't have much left. It would be

great if I won the lottery. There was one job that might have had something, but I would have to commute, and I hate that.

Therapist: This has been going on for a long time. You no longer have signs or symptoms of depression, so the current medication seems right. I think your problem is demoralization. That's a condition in which a person is convinced that his or her efforts will not succeed, so the person does nothing. The only way out is to begin doing things—anything. Small steps lead to small successes. It's a rehabilitation approach. It affects self-esteem and confidence. (***The therapist names, explains, and gives advice.***)

# Expanding the Patient's Awareness

Our efforts to make the patient aware of thoughts or feelings he or she had not been aware of are *clarification, confrontation,* and *interpretation.*

## Clarification

*Clarification* is summarizing, paraphrasing, or organizing what the patient has said. Often, clarification simply demonstrates that the therapist is attentive and is processing what he or she hears. Clarification is an awareness-expanding intervention. Whether in psychotherapy or not, people say things without appreciating the significance of what they have said. In the next dialogue, the therapist clarifies through summarizing:

Patient: I can't get things done. I have to sell the house, but first I have to get some things fixed, and I don't do it. My ex-wife keeps harassing me with court papers about unpaid child support. I think the medication is working, but it takes the edge off my creativity. She's relentless. I'm bipolar. Don't they have to take that into account? My car broke down again, too.

Therapist: It sounds like you're saying that you're overwhelmed.

## Confrontation

As a technical term, *confrontation* does not imply hostility or aggression. *Confrontation* means bringing to the patient's attention a pattern of behavior, ideas, or feelings he or she has not recognized or has avoided. In the following continuation of the dialogue in "Clarification," the therapist uses confrontation:

Patient 1: I'm living alone in that big house. If I sell it, I can get a smaller place and have money left over, but I just don't do anything. I'm so depressed.

> Therapist 1: It sounds like you are avoiding doing the one thing that would provide you enough money to pay your bills and give your ex-wife what she wants. (***The therapist knows that** depression **is a universally used word and that the patient who says, "I'm depressed" does not necessarily meet the criteria for any depressive disorder.***)

In the early years of psychotherapy, sexual feelings were often unknown to the patient until the psychotherapist helped the patient to become aware of them. Anger is often outside awareness. The hidden anger may be directed toward authority figures, people who are more successful, those who are manipulative, or those who are dependent and passive. Anger may be the emotional response to paranoid ideation. The discovery of anger does not always clear the air.

What are some other feelings that are often kept out of awareness? Excessive dependence on another person is often associated with resentment. Resentment is related to anger—resentment of parents, children, partners, co-workers. Resentment has been described as a negative emotion, and it is often accompanied by guilt or shame. Grief may be a hidden emotion for those who do not grieve the death of someone close. After stabilization with atypical antipsychotics, schizophrenic individuals whose lives have long been disrupted may be able to grieve for the years they have lost and grieve over the suffering they have caused. For other individuals, feelings of intimacy and caring are kept out of awareness. Vulnerability scares some so much that they push it out of their minds. The list can go on and on.

To simply name the feeling and move on is a supportive technique. When we are exploring a patient's hitherto unexamined feelings and assumptions, we seek to learn of other, related instances of whatever we have discovered or to talk about the implications of the discovery, to understand the basis for it, and ultimately, to determine what is to be done about it.

## Interpretation

There is no agreed-on definition of *interpretation*. Many authors use the term to characterize any proffered explanation of "the meaning of the patient's thoughts or the intent of his behavior" (Othmer and Othmer 1994, p. 87). Others limit the term to a linking of current feelings, thoughts, or behaviors with events of the past or the relationship with the therapist. Linking all three elements is important for achieving the objectives of expressive psychotherapy. In supportive psychotherapy, patient–therapist linkages are generally made only when necessary to avoid disruption of treatment.

## Conclusion

Supportive techniques can be enumerated and mastered. With practice, these techniques can be applied usefully in many situations. More lengthy elaboration of techniques can be found in a handful of books. Especially useful are the works by Pinsker (1997), Wachtel (1993), Winston and Winston (2002), Rockland (1989), and Novalis et al. (1993).

Guidance about understanding the patient can be found in many thousands of books on psychodynamics and psychotherapy written in the last 75 years, and in literature of the last 500 years.

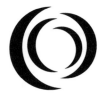

# 4

# Assessment, Case Formulation, Goal Setting, and Outcome Research

## Assessment

The process of evaluation and case formulation is an essential element of all psychotherapeutic approaches. A central objective of the assessment process is to diagnose the patient's illness and describe the problems so that the patient can be treated appropriately. Another important objective of the evaluation process is to establish a therapeutic relationship, which can further the patient's interest in and commitment to psychotherapy. A thorough evaluation should help the clinician to select the appropriate treatment approach. The treatment plan should be individualized to meet the needs and goals of the patient.

The psychotherapy/psychopathology continuum discussed in Chapter 1, "Basic Principles of Supportive Psychotherapy," is a useful way of thinking about the evaluation process. When a therapist meets a patient for the first time, the therapist generally does not know the extent of the patient's impairment, psychopathology, or strengths. Therefore, the initial interview should begin with the therapist's attempting to understand why the patient has come for treatment. All patients should have a thorough evaluation of current problems and past history. However, the technical approach will vary: a more supportive one for patients on the left side of the continuum (higher levels of psychopathology) and a more expressive one for patients on the right side of the continuum (lower levels of psychopathology). If it becomes clear that the patient has significant psychopathology, the therapist may have to quickly move into a more supportive mode. The degree of disturbance encountered during the initial interview will determine how the clinician proceeds in that interview.

The supportive-expressive psychotherapy continuum concept is the traditional way of thinking about dynamic psychotherapy. In this conceptualization, supportive psychotherapy is indicated for patients with high levels of psychopathology, whereas expressive psychotherapy is better suited for healthier patients. However, in our clinical and research work, we have found that supportive and expressive psychotherapies produce similar results in patients across the psychopathology continuum (see "Outcome Research" later in this chapter). The efficacy of supportive psychotherapy in higher-functioning patients is especially enhanced when expressive and cognitive-behavioral techniques are integrated into a supportive approach (Winston and Winston 2002). Therefore, supportive psychotherapy is indicated for a wide variety of disorders across the psychopathology continuum (see Chapter 5, "General Framework of Supportive Psychotherapy," for a full discussion of inclusion and exclusion criteria for supportive psychotherapy).

The evaluation should be comprehensive and, if possible, should be completed during an extended first session of at least 60 minutes. At the end of the evaluation, the therapist should understand the patient's problems, interpersonal relationships, everyday functioning, and psychological structure. The evaluation interview should not be a series of questions and answers but should be more of an exploration of the patient's life. The interview should be therapeutic, to help motivate the patient for treatment and promote the therapeutic alliance. In a supportive approach, making an evaluation therapeutic generally involves use of trial therapy (Davanloo 1980; Laikin et al. 1991), encompassing appropriate interventions such as clarification and confrontation in an empathic manner.

The evaluation should begin with an exploration of the patient's presenting problems or areas of disturbance. Presenting problems may include symptoms, relationship and self difficulties, work or school issues, medical problems, and substance abuse issues. Generally, symptoms should be explored first so that the clinician is informed about the extent of the patient's psychopathology. Exploring symptoms first is also helpful to the patient because symptoms are what patients care about. Information about symptoms will enable the clinician to adjust the evaluation interview to the patient's level of psychopathology. When significant impairment exists, the interview should be more supportive, whereas with more cognitively intact patients, the interviewer can use an exploratory approach. With some patients, this distinction will be clear from the start, particularly if the patient has a loss of reality testing. With other patients, the extent of psychopathology may not be as readily discernible, so it may take more time to make this determination.

After the presenting problems have been clearly delineated, the therapist should explore the patient's history. This exploration can be done in many ways but should be systematic and should cover relationships with parents, other caretakers, siblings, grandparents, and other people in the patient's life and household; descriptions of these individuals should also be obtained. Important issues to inquire about include trauma, separation and loss, medical problems and psychiatric illness (in the patient and first-degree relatives), geographic moves, family belief systems, school history, sexual development and experiences, identity issues, and financial matters. Past psychiatric treatment, including psychotherapy and pharmacotherapy, should be explored, as should the patient's response to the therapist, because this knowledge can alert the therapist to potential problems in the therapeutic alliance.

As soon as the therapist determines that the patient should be treated with supportive psychotherapy, the evaluation interview should promote the objectives of supportive psychotherapy: to ameliorate symptoms and to maintain, restore, or improve self-esteem, adaptive skills, and ego or psychological functions (Pinsker et al. 1991).

A useful method of conceptualizing dynamic psychotherapy, which encompasses both supportive and expressive approaches, involves the triangles of conflict and person. The focus of the triangle of conflict (Freud 1926/1959; Malan 1979) (Figure 4–1) is on wishes, needs, and feelings that are warded off by defenses and anxiety. In this model, a therapist who is pursuing a patient's feeling is at the wish/need/feeling point of the triangle. As is often the case, the patient may respond defensively to the exploration of feeling. Defense is the second point of the triangle. The patient also may respond with anxiety because of fear of the conflicted feeling. Anxiety is the third point of this triangle.

In the triangle of the person (Malan 1979; Menninger 1958) (Figure 4–2), the three points all relate to people and include individuals in the patient's current life and past life and the therapist or transference figure. In expressive or exploratory psychotherapy, the therapist tends to

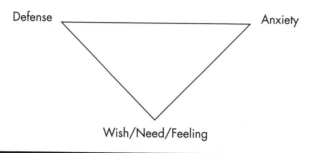

**Figure 4–1.** Triangle of conflict.

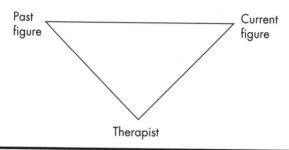

**Figure 4–2.** Triangle of person.

work on conflict situations using the triangles to explore wishes, needs, and feelings that the patient may have in relation to an important person in his or her life. When defenses interfere with exploration, they are addressed. Present and past issues are addressed, and the transference relationship and its exploration are emphasized.

In supportive psychotherapy, the triangles of conflict and person are used differently. In the triangle of conflict, feelings generally are not pursued, anxiety is diminished, and defenses are strengthened. In the triangle of the person, the real relationship with the therapist is emphasized, and the therapist works primarily on present persons and current issues in the patient's life.

The following vignette from an initial evaluation session illustrates a supportive evaluation.

## Case Vignette: Supportive Evaluation

Mary, a 42-year-old woman, was referred by her primary care physician because of depression, beginning at age 24, and a number of other problems. She recently went through a divorce and is having great difficulty finding a job. She has a history of multiple episodes of depression and was hospitalized once for suicidal depression.

> Therapist: As you know, Dr. Perry suggested you see me for an evaluation. Can you tell me what the problem is?
>
> Mary: I just don't feel right. I don't know....I can't seem to get anything done. (***Responds in a vague manner that could be defensive or a sign of disorganization***)
>
> Therapist: So you don't feel right and can't get anything done and seem at a loss. (***Responds with a supportive clarification that helps Mary to focus on the question at hand***)
>
> Mary: Yes, I just sit around...can't get started...everything's a mess. I just feel bad. [*becomes tearful*]

The therapist recognizes that the patient may be depressed and asks a series of questions to determine whether the patient is depressed and the extent of the depression.

- Have you been feeling down? Have you been crying or feeling tearful?
- What is your energy level like? Have you been tired a lot?
- Are you anxious, fearful, jumpy?
- What about your sleep patterns? Are you having problems falling asleep or are you sleeping too much?
- How is your appetite? Are you losing or gaining weight?
- Are you able to take care of your daily tasks at home and at work?
- Are you maintaining your social relationships? Do you find pleasure in your life? Do you go out?
- What is your attitude about the future? Do you feel hopeful?
- Do you feel life is not worth living? Do you have thoughts of hurting yourself? Plans to hurt yourself? Have you tried to hurt yourself?
- Are you able to have sexual relations? Is sex pleasurable?

Mary responds that for the past 2 months, she has been consistently downhearted, tearful, fatigued, and pessimistic about the future and has had difficulty concentrating. She has trouble falling asleep, consistently awakens during early morning hours, and is unable to go back to sleep. Her appetite is poor, and she has lost approximately 10 pounds in the past 2 weeks. She is preoccupied with death and has thoughts of killing herself but no defined plan. She rarely goes out, nothing gives her pleasure or satisfaction, and she has no sexual desire or interest. She has never had a manic or hypomanic episode. Mary had her first episode of depression when she was 24 years old and was hospitalized in her mid-30s for suicidal depression. In the past, she was treated with antidepressants. During her last episode, she was treated with paroxetine. Mary stopped taking her medication 6 months ago.

The therapist recognizes that the patient is in the midst of a major depressive episode and has some cognitive difficulties. This level of psychopathology places Mary on the left side of the continuum, which indicates that the therapist should continue the evaluation in a supportive mode.

> Therapist: From what you've told me, it seems you're depressed now and have been depressed several times in the past. What you've been experiencing—tearfulness, fatigue, difficulty concentrating, sleep problems, feeling bad about yourself, and having trouble with day-to-day tasks of living—are all symptoms of depression.

The therapist has begun to educate the patient about her depression. Education is important in all forms of psychotherapy but especially in supportive treatment. Education provides the patient with knowledge about his or her difficulties and also demonstrates the therapist's interest and understanding, thereby promoting the therapeutic alliance.

Next, the therapist explores how the current episode of depression began:

> Mary: I knew I was feeling down, but so many things were bothering me...
>
> Therapist: Let's see if we can understand what brought on this depression. You've been severely depressed for 2 months, is that right? (**Begins to focus on possible precipitants of Mary's depression**)
>
> Mary: Yes, that's right....I really started to feel terrible 2 months ago. It was September...but I don't think I felt well before that...maybe for at least a year.
>
> Therapist: Can you recall...did anything significant happen in your life that might have caused you to feel so down? (**Continues to focus**)
>
> Mary [long pause]: I don't know. [tearful] (**Is verbally defensive, but underlying affect breaks through**)
>
> Therapist: I can see this is hard for you. (**Responds in an empathic manner to Mary's tearfulness**)
>
> Mary: Well, something did happen. I found out that Edward—my husband—was involved with a woman who worked with him. [weeping] [long pause] I don't like to talk about this. (**Begins to reveal important material that may have contributed to the onset of the depression**)
>
> Therapist: Many people would find it difficult. (**Responds in a supportive manner to let Mary know that her reluctance to talk about a difficult emotional situation is not unusual**)
>
> Mary: I couldn't believe it. We had been together for 14 years....I thought things were good. He betrayed me. I still can't believe it!

Therapist: How awful for you. (**Responds in an empathic manner to continue to support Mary**)

Mary [*begins to sob*]: As soon as I found out, I stopped going to my job. I knew I couldn't just go on as usual. (**Indicates that her husband's infidelity and leaving her led to a series of negative behaviors**)

Therapist: What prevented you from going to work?

Mary: Um…I don't know.…I just didn't have the energy.…I felt like a failure. I just couldn't face anyone. I didn't want anyone to know.…Who knows what they would say about me.

It appears that the discovery of her husband's infidelity played a major role in the onset of Mary's current depression. Her inability to continue to work, coupled with concern about what others would think, reflects an adaptive failure and a loss of self-esteem. The thought that others would think of her as a failure indicates that she has negative thoughts (automatic thoughts) about herself, which she attributes to others.

Therapist: What do you believe your co-workers would say or think about you? (**Begins to explore Mary's automatic thinking**)

Mary: That Edward thought I'm a loser.

Therapist: How is that?

Mary: Well, that I bothered him. I called him a lot…whenever I needed help or felt lonely, even though I was at work and he was at work. He used to get angry. "What are you always calling me for? Can't you think things through for yourself?"

Therapist: How did you react to that?

Mary: I got more upset. I began to feel that I was incompetent. (**Articulates an automatic thought**)

Therapist: So you thought of yourself as incompetent. But is that really true? Can you give me an example of this? (**First clarifies Mary's automatic thought and begins to question her negative thinking; then asks for a concrete example. Remaining at an abstract or general level promotes vagueness and loss of focus.**)

Mary: Well, once I accidentally banged my head into something; it was really bad. It was during lunch hour, and I began to bleed. I was a mess.…I knew I needed stitches, so I called my husband, hoping he would come with me to the doctor. But he said, "I'm busy. Take care of it yourself. What are you—helpless?" And then I did feel helpless, like I couldn't do anything for myself. (**Provides a clear interpersonal example**)

Therapist: So you were bleeding and feeling you needed your husband to help you, and instead he refused to help and in fact put you down. I'm wondering if this incident and others like it have given you the idea that you're incompetent? (**Provides a clarification of Mary's description and conclusion**)

Mary: Well…yeah.

Therapist: I don't know if you would agree with me, but most people would call on someone close to them for help. It seems to me that you drew an erroneous conclusion about yourself. I wonder if this kind of pattern has been with you for a long time?

The therapist has elicited a concrete example of an interaction with the patient's husband, an interaction that led the patient to think of herself as incompetent and helpless. This way of thinking is an example of automatic thoughts, which are quite common in depression. Mary's thinking patterns would constitute an important area on which to concentrate in supportive therapy for this type of disorder. In this instance, the therapist has attempted to point out that Mary's negative thinking was faulty, but the therapist has done so in a supportive manner by asking if Mary agreed. In subsequent sessions, the therapist should help the patient to test her automatic thoughts herself.

The therapist then goes on to explore the patient's relationship with Edward and the history of their marriage. Mary believed that her relationship with Edward was fine. He was helpful to her in all ways. He made most of the decisions in their marriage, and Mary relied on him for reassurance and support. She called him many times each day and had difficulty managing by herself when he went away on business trips. Edward left Mary 4 months after her discovery of his infidelity, and they were divorced approximately 1 month before she became clinically depressed.

For more than 20 years, Mary worked as a paralegal in a large law firm. Although she was a valued employee and could be relied on to get the job done, her relationship with co-workers was conflictual. She was often angry with them and critical of them. Approximately 3 years ago, she gave up her job as a paralegal because she felt overwhelmed, and she began to work in various temporary positions lasting 2–3 weeks at a time. She explained that life was easier working part-time, without conflicts or responsibilities at the end of the day.

Mary is the youngest of three sisters and is considered the baby of the family. Her sisters, 10 and 15 years her senior, are successful and are often critical of Mary's lack of ambition. Mary's mother was 41 and her father 43 years old when she was born. Her mother considered having an abortion when she was pregnant with Mary. The patient was often sick as a child, and her mother was overprotective, worrying a great deal about her health and safety. Mary's father worked long hours and had limited interaction with his daughter. Despite his unavailability, Mary has positive memories of the time they did spend together. She recalls hearing him return home after work late in the evenings and feeling comforted by the sound of his footsteps. When Mary was 14 years old, her father died suddenly of a heart attack. She has only vague memories surrounding his death but remembers that her mother became unavailable and was increasingly critical of her at that time.

The patient is in the throes of a major depressive episode and has had four previous major depressive episodes, as well as a milder, chronic depression for most of her life. Serious difficulties in the interpersonal sphere, as well as personality problems, limit her ability to function. The therapist, a psychiatrist, concluded that Mary would benefit from medication and a supportive approach employing cognitive-behavioral techniques. The therapist explained how both approaches—medication and psychotherapy—would be helpful in treating Mary's depression, anxiety, and problems in day-to-day functioning. The patient agreed with these immediate treatment goals and stated that she thought the medication and psychotherapy were worth a try. An explanation was given about when the medication would begin to work and would have maximum effect. In addition, possible side effects of the medication were discussed.

### Diagnostic Evaluation

- *Axis I:* Major depressive disorder, recurrent
- *Axis II:* Dependent personality disorder
- *Axis III:* None
- *Axis IV:* Loss of husband
- *Axis V:* Global Assessment of Functioning=55

## Case Formulation

For each patient, the treatment approach should be based on the central issues emerging from the assessment and case formulation. Case formulation depends on an accurate and thorough assessment of the patient. The case formulation is an explanation of the patient's symptoms and psychosocial functioning. The therapist's formulation governs his or her interventions as well as which issues in the patient–therapist dialogue are selected for attention. Having a sense of the underlying issues at the start enhances the therapist's ability to respond empathically. At the same time, empathy for the patient helps the therapist to guide and plan therapy effectively. The initial formulation is tentative and must be modified as more is learned about the patient during the course of psychotherapy. The DSM diagnosis is important. It is an element of the formulation but by no means the whole story. It does not illuminate an individual's adaptive or maladaptive characteristics, such as disappointments, the capacity for relationships, and how the individual thinks about and interprets life's events. Nor does the diagnosis explain the unique life history of an individual. The DSM diagnosis alone does not explain the patient or the problem.

The following case formulation approaches are derived from psychoanalytic, interpersonal, relational, and cognitive-behavioral approaches. Supportive psychotherapy uses elements of all these therapies but differs in how these elements are used. For example, a patient's conflict may be clearly understood and formulated by the therapist but never or only partially explored in psychotherapy. Although these approaches have always been described separately, a great deal of overlap exists, so there is some repetition in the descriptions.

## Structural Approach

A structural case formulation attempts to capture the relatively fixed characteristics of an individual's personality, which is understood within a functional context (in contrast with dynamic and genetic approaches, which are more content based). Assessment of an individual's strengths and weaknesses and overall level of psychopathology helps determine the clinician's choice of technical approaches. A thorough structural assessment enables the clinician to determine with some degree of accuracy where to place the patient on the psychopathological–psychological structure continuum (see Chapter 1, "Basic Principles of Supportive Psychotherapy," for a discussion of this continuum).

Structural functions have been grouped together using Freud's (1923/1961) structural approach of id, ego, and superego. These agencies refer to the inner life of the patient. The following description of psychological or ego functions is based on the work of Beres (1956) and Bellak (1958). These categories are not mutually exclusive; there is a great deal of overlap.

**Relation to reality.** Beres and Bellak described reality testing and sense of reality as major components of relation to reality (Bellak 1958; Beres 1956). The term reality testing describes an individual's ability to assess reality. Reality testing is impaired in the presence of faulty judgment and is grossly disturbed in the presence of hallucinations or delusions. _Sense of reality_ relates to a person's ability to distinguish self from other; presence of this ability indicates a stable and cohesive body image. Examples of disturbances in this function are depersonalization, derealization, and identity problems.

Disturbances in relation to reality indicate significant structural problems that place the patient on the left side of the psychopathological-psychological structure continuum, and such disturbances should point the clinician in the direction of a more supportive approach. Impaired relation to reality is a key indicator of structural deficits and should always be thoroughly explored.

**Object relations.** Object relations refers to a person's capacity to relate in a meaningful way to significant individuals in his or her life. The function includes the ability to form intimate relationships, tolerate separation and loss, and maintain independence and autonomy. It also involves the sense of self and the ability to form a cohesive and stable self-image without diminishing or overidealizing self or other.

A patient's relationships with others form the foundation of the psychological functions constituting the structural approach. In all forms of psychotherapy, evaluation of object relations is central in determining a patient's placement on the psychopathological–psychological structure continuum. Patients who are withdrawn and not interested in others or who have narcissistic, highly dependent, or chaotic relationships generally require a more supportive approach and therefore are on the left side of the continuum. Individuals who have had at least one meaningful give-and-take relationship tend to be on the right side of the continuum.

**Affects, impulse control, and defenses.** Affects are complex psycho-physiological states composed of subjective feelings and physiological accompaniments such as crying, blushing, sweating, posture, facial expression, and tone of voice. The range of affects includes excitement, joy, surprise, fear, anger, rage, irritation, anguish, shame, humiliation, sadness, and depression. The individual's ability to experience a wide range of affects at some depth and how well the individual differentiates between affects (as opposed to lumping them into a single feeling such as primitive rage) need to be assessed. Is there a wide variety and range of affects, and is the individual able to tolerate love, anger, joy, sadness, or humiliation? What are the predominant affects (Friedman and Lister 1987), and how regularly are they invoked?

The capacity to *control impulses* and to modulate affect in an adaptive manner indicates a well-functioning defensive structure. When impulse control is faulty, the individual may engage in socially unacceptable behavior, such as physically or verbally lashing out at others or making inappropriate demands. The ability to delay gratification and to tolerate frustration is another important aspect of impulse control.

*Defenses* mediate between a person's wishes, needs, and feelings and both internal prohibitions and the external world. Individuals tend to use the same kinds of behavior as patterned responses in reaction to perceived danger, difficult situations, or painful affects. Defenses are conceptualized as having both a developmental and a hierarchical organization. Three levels of defenses have been described: immature, intermediate, and mature. Some immature defenses are projection, hypochondriasis, acting out, sarcasm, and avoidance. Intermediate defenses include forgetting, intellectualization, displacement, and rationalization. Among the mature defenses are altruism, anticipation, suppression, sublimation, and humor (Vaillant 1977, 1986). Primitive defenses, poor impulse control, severe affective instability, and shallow affect are indicators of structural deficits that place an individual on the left side of the continuum and suggest the need for a more supportive approach.

**Thought processes.** The ability to think clearly, logically, and abstractly should be assessed. High levels of primary process or primitive thinking are a good indicator of severe psychopathology. Significant limitations in the ability to think logically suggest the need for a more supportive approach as opposed to an exploratory one. Dysfunctional and automatic thoughts should be identified so that cognitive-behavioral approaches can be applied.

**Autonomous functions.** Autonomous functions—perception, intention, intelligence, language, and motor development—are believed to develop in a relatively conflict-free manner (Hartmann 1939/1958). Although these functions generally are not impaired in patients on the right side of the psychopathological/psychological structure continuum, the functions can be affected in patients with significant psychopathology.

**Synthetic function.** The synthetic function (Nunberg 1931) is the ability to organize oneself and the world in a productive manner. It is the psychological ability to form a cohesive whole, or gestalt, by putting together the other functions and organizing them, so that one can function in a harmonious and integrated way.

**Conscience, morals, and ideals.** Conscience, morals, and ideals derive from internalization of aspects of parental figures and social mores. Freud (1926/1959) conceptualized these elements as aspects of the superego. Severe impairments in these functions can interfere with the patient–therapist relationship. For instance, if a patient is not truthful with the therapist, achieving success in psychotherapy may be difficult.

## Case Vignette: Structural Case Formulation

The following vignette provides the basis for a structural case formulation:

> Bert, a 24-year-old man with panic disorder, has developed the belief that his co-workers are saying derogatory things about him and want to hurt him physically. His relationships are characterized by an absence of concern for self or others, and this lack of concern often puts him at risk. He uses women to satisfy his sexual needs, abruptly leaving them, giving untruthful excuses. At times he becomes enraged with and is physically abusive toward them. His aggressive and violent behavior evokes fears of retaliation. He both uses and sells drugs. The patient has a history of beginning schools and jobs and then quitting them when he encounters difficulties, blaming others for his failures.

This vignette illustrates a number of structural deficits. The patient has impaired reality testing, consisting of ideas about others talking and plotting against him. His adaptive skills are poor, as demonstrated by his inability to work or to complete school. Relationships are conducted on a need-satisfying basis, without concern for others. Bert is often sadistic but then becomes self-defeating and self-punishing. He exhibits impaired frustration tolerance and poorly controlled impulses, and his displays of rage may indicate a limited repertoire of affective responses. He uses immature defense such as projection, acting out, and denial.

## Genetic Approach

The genetic area of case formulation involves exploration of early development and life events that may help to explain an individual's current situation. Genetics are the genesis of the dynamics. Life presents many challenges, conflicts, and crises. These can be traumatic, depending on their severity, the developmental stage of the child, and the quality of his or her support system. Events or conditions such as the loss of a significant person, separation, abuse, the birth of a sibling, birth defects and developmental deficits, learning problems, illness, surgery, and substance abuse need to be considered as important in a child's development. A single event can have a traumatic effect on an individual, although often it is the day-to-day negative experiences that lead to significant conflict, psychopathology, and characterological problems. Examples of day-to-day events are constant criticism, devaluing, abusive behavior, parental conflict, and significant psychiatric problems. The genetic approach follows the development of the child from birth to late adolescence and/or early adulthood.

An example of a persistent difficulty or traumatic situation is the experience of a young boy growing up with a violent alcoholic father who is demeaning and at times physically abusive. Persistent trauma such as that caused by unresponsiveness of a parent may be more subtle and difficult to evaluate. For instance, a narcissistic mother may use her daughter for her own self-enhancement. She may ignore her child's real qualities, demanding behavior the child is either unable to deliver or can deliver only at considerable cost to herself.

## Dynamic Approach

The dynamic approach concerns itself with mental and/or emotional tensions that may be conscious or unconscious. The approach focuses on conflicting wishes, needs, or feelings, and on their meanings. In a conflict situation, an individual wards off or defends against wishes, needs, or feelings. The dynamic approach highlights the content of an individual's current conflicts and relates it to a primary lifelong or core conflict (S. Perry et al. 1987).

Dynamic case formulation is concerned with meaning and content; in contrast, structural case formulation is based on an individual's relatively fixed characteristics and functioning. The dynamic approach focuses on current conflicts, whereas the genetic approach highlights a person's developmental history and describes childhood and adolescent traumas and conflicts and their possible meanings. Childhood conflicts tend to be revived and relived in adult life.

A useful approach to understanding the dynamics of an individual, particularly the core conflict, involves mapping the central relationship patterns. An understanding of these patterns requires exploration of three aspects of interpersonal interactions: 1) what the person wants from others, 2) how others react to the person, and 3) how the person responds to others' reactions. These categories form the basis of the core conflictual relationship theme (CCRT) method, an approach that relies on "narratives, called relationship episodes, that patients typically tell and sometimes even enact during their psychotherapy session" (Luborsky and Crits-Christoph 1990, p. 15). The CCRT is composed of the patient's wishes or needs of others and how others respond (their actual responses as well as their responses from the patient's perspective). Understanding and using the CCRT method provides the clinician with a central organizing focus. The CCRT method can be used differentially with patients according to their position on the continuum.

### Case Vignette: Dynamic Case Formulation

The following vignette illustrates a dynamic conflict as well as its genetic or historical basis:

> Tim is a passive 48-year-old man whose father has become increasingly debilitated and demanding, a state made worse by early signs of dementia. His father often telephones with complaints and demands, even though Tim has been consistently helpful. After these calls, Tim finds himself wishing that his father appreciated him. He becomes anxiety ridden and often is angry with his wife and friends, later feeling guilty about his behavior. At work, he has become increasingly anxious and perfectionistic, and he worries that his boss dislikes him and will criticize him.

The dynamic explanation is that Tim has ambivalent feelings toward his father, consisting of anger and possibly a wish for his father to die, combined with positive feelings based on earlier experiences. He becomes anxious and defends against these feelings or wishes by displacing the anger he feels toward his father onto his wife and friends. The anxiety serves as a signal of unacceptable feelings. His boss is viewed as an authority figure and has become linked with his father, who is both loved and hated. In general, Tim is passive and avoids confrontation. He fears making a mistake and being humiliated. According to the CCRT method, Tim's wish to be appreciated by his father can be identified. The response of the other is lack of appreciation combined with hostility, and the response of the self is displacement of anger onto Tim's wife and friends and feeling unappreciated. The genetic basis of Tim's current conflict is related to his experiencing his father as being both highly critical, and concerned and loving to him when he was a youngster. This early experience resulted in mixed feelings toward his father, consisting of love and rage with accompanying anxiety, guilt, and lack of assertiveness.

## Cognitive-Behavioral Approach

The cognitive-behavioral approach addresses an individual's underlying psychological structure and the content of his or her thoughts. It is believed that the way in which an individual experiences environmental events and responds to them is greatly determined by cognitive processes. Cognitive theory postulates that problems develop from the activation of underlying core beliefs by stressful life events. Prior experience determines how an individual perceives an event, the meaning he or she assigns to it, whether the event is attended to or remembered, and whether it affects the individual's future functioning (note the similarity to genetic and dynamic formulations).

Although case formulation has not been widely used in cognitive-behavioral therapy, models have been developed that are helpful in assessing an individual's problems in cognition (Persons 1989, 1993). Cognitive-behavioral therapy is initially directed at automatic thoughts, which are based on core beliefs or negative schemas. Overt and underlying beliefs are closely linked and are expressed as thoughts, behaviors, and moods. Core beliefs are addressed later in the course of therapy. The cognitive-behavioral case formulation model has the following eight components (Tompkins 1996):

1. Problem list (including automatic thoughts)
2. Core beliefs
3. Conditional beliefs
4. Origins
5. Precipitants and activating situations
6. Working hypothesis
7. Predicted obstacles to treatment
8. Treatment plan

The description of Tim (see "Case Vignette: Dynamic Case Formulation" in the previous section) will be used to illustrate these eight components and cognitive-behavioral case formulation.

The *problem list* is a complete list of the patient's difficulties and presenting complaints. It includes the dysfunctional thinking responsible for the maladaptive behavior and disturbed mood. Tim's mood problems are anxiety, anger, and feelings of guilt. His problematic behavior is his inappropriate rage at his wife and friends. His automatic thoughts ("I am flawed" and "I will make mistakes and be humiliated") lead to passivity and lack of assertiveness.

Core beliefs are hypotheses about the patient's self-schemas and views of others and the world. Tim's core belief is a pervasive sense that he cannot do anything right. This belief makes him especially vulnerable to the opinions of others and to conditional (if-then) beliefs, which can increase his anxiety. An example of a conditional belief is the belief that if one makes a mistake, others will be very critical. The origins of core beliefs are early experiences, generally involving parents or parental figures. Tim's core beliefs appear to have derived from his relationship with his overly critical father.

Core beliefs are generally *activated by situations or events* that are stressful or problematic for the patient. The deteriorating health of the patient's father precipitated Tim's current difficulty and brought him into treatment.

The *working hypothesis* forms the core of the cognitive-behavioral case formulation and incorporates the problem list, the core beliefs, and the activating events. Tim's anxiety, anger, guilt, passivity, and lack of assertiveness are based on his core beliefs that he cannot do anything right and that if he makes a mistake, others will be very critical of him. These problems and core beliefs were activated or made worse by his father's dementia.

*Obstacles to treatment* should be anticipated if possible. Obstacles in Tim's case might be reflected in the patient–therapist relationship. Fear of criticism can emerge in relation to the therapist and lead to increased patient passivity in the treatment situation. Tim may be reluctant to complete homework assignments because he fears that the therapist will be critical.

A well-thought-out and comprehensive *treatment plan* should emerge from the case formulation. This plan should include goals and the types of interventions to be used.

## The Four Approaches Compared and Applied

There are a number of similarities between the four discussed case formulation approaches in dynamic (supportive and expressive) and cognitive-behavioral therapies. The concept of core beliefs and their origins is similar to the idea of the genetic case formulation, which provides the origins of structural and dynamic factors. The notion of activating events in cognitive-behavioral therapy also is analogous to the precipitation of genetic and dynamic conflicts. Obstacles to treatment often relate to the therapeutic relationship, and thus the concept of obstacles is similar in genetic and dynamic approaches. Cognitive-behavioral therapy adds a different dimension to case formulation and the treatment approach, particularly when thinking problems are present. Dynamic and genetic approaches do not involve a major focus on thinking, but the structural approach does evaluate an individual's thought processes.

Following are case formulations and diagnostic assessments of Mary, the patient evaluated in "Case Vignette: Supportive Evaluation" near the beginning of the chapter.

### Structural Approach

Mary is an intelligent woman with limited insight and judgment. Although her reality testing is intact, her adaptive skills are impaired. She has difficulty functioning, caring for herself, and working. Her object relations are on a need-satisfying level. Mary has low self-esteem, a result of early experiences with her mother and sisters and more recent experiences with her husband. Her depression has intensified her feelings of inadequacy. The defenses Mary uses are at the immature level and consist of avoidance, denial, and projection. Predominant affects are sadness and anger. Mary has many negative thoughts about herself and is somewhat impulsive.

## Genetic Approach

Mary is the youngest of three girls born to older parents. Her parents did not expect a third child, and her mother considered aborting the pregnancy. Mary grew up with a sense of not being wanted by her mother. Mary felt she was the least favored child compared with her sisters, who were admired by their mother for their intelligence and beauty. Her mother's attitude toward her interfered with her development of a positive self-image, resulting in faltering self-esteem. When Mary was 14 years old, her father—with whom she had a predominantly positive relationship—suddenly died. At that time, her mother became less available and was more critical of Mary. The death of her father, who had been a source of comfort during adolescence, may have added to her impaired self-esteem and her neediness.

## Dynamic Approach

Mary is a needy, dependent woman who wishes to be cared for. The patient's core conflict revolves around her wish to be wanted and cared for by others (mother and husband). When the response of others is to abandon her (father's death), criticize her, or favor others (sisters and husband's lover), she becomes depressed and withdrawn, with diminished self-esteem. Her wish to be cared for is an expression of her need to feel she has a right to exist.

## Cognitive-Behavioral Approach

Mary's problems include depression, interpersonal difficulties with her husband and co-workers, and an inability to maintain day-to-day functioning. Her automatic thoughts are "I can't do anything right" and "I need someone to care for me." These automatic thoughts are based on Mary's core beliefs that she is worthless, a failure, and in need of constant support, without which she cannot function. The origins of her core beliefs are her mother's and sisters' view that she was weak, sickly, and not as capable as her sisters.

Precipitants of and activating situations for Mary's difficulties are the loss of her husband and the discontinuation of her medication for previous depression. The obstacles to treatment are Mary's severe neediness and her fear that the therapist will view her as inadequate.

## Goal Setting

For patients requiring supportive psychotherapy, organizing goals should be amelioration of symptoms and improvement and enhancement of adaptation, self-esteem, and overall functioning. Setting goals in psychotherapy is important in guiding the treatment, because both therapist and patient must agree on the objectives of treatment. The goals set within the first few sessions should be viewed as preliminary and open to change. Both immediate objectives for each session and ultimate goals (Parloff 1967) for treatment should be considered. An immediate in-session objective may be to develop a mutually agreed-on plan for helping Mary return to work within a week. An ultimate goal would be to promote job stability and improve relationships with co-workers.

Clearly outlined goals help motivate patients and promote the therapeutic alliance as patient and therapist work toward a common end. The goals of treatment should be derived from the patient's problem areas so that motivation to change will be enhanced and will promote therapeutic clarity.

The goals of therapy should generally be the patient's. In the event of disagreement on goals, the therapist enters into an exploration of the problem. In the case of Mary, one of the mutually agreed-on goals was to resolve her depression and to prevent future episodes of depression. However, during Mary's previous episodes of depression, she stopped taking her medication when she was no longer depressed. It would be important for Mary to maintain the goal of continuing her medication, to help prevent future depressive episodes. Exploring the reasons she stopped taking her medication, and educating her about the risks of discontinuing, eventually led to obtaining her agreement with this treatment goal.

It is important to set realistic goals, especially with patients who have severe psychopathology. Some patients may have grandiose fantasies or magical wishes that will need to be modified. Mary had the unrealistic expectation that her husband would return to her, which she thought would solve her problems.

Treatment goals should never be regarded as fixed and unchangeable. For example, once Mary's depression is resolved, she may want help with expanding her social network and improving her interpersonal relationships.

# Outcome Research

There have been a limited number of controlled clinical trials of supportive psychotherapy. In this section, we present some early uncontrolled studies and some more recent controlled trials that bear on the efficacy of supportive psychotherapy.

## Menninger Psychotherapy Research Project

The psychotherapy research project of the Menninger Foundation was an important early study comparing supportive and expressive psychotherapy with psychoanalysis. Wallerstein and co-workers (Wallerstein 1986, 1989) studied the treatment, clinical course, and posttreatment follow-up of 42 inpatients at the Menninger Foundation. Findings included the following: psychoanalysis produced more limited outcomes than predicted, whereas psychotherapy including supportive therapy often achieved more than predicted; all the treatments became more supportive during the course of therapy, and supportive interventions accounted for more of the change in outcome. This study took a naturalistic approach, without control subjects or random assignment of subjects, but was noteworthy in calling attention to the possible efficacy of supportive psychotherapy.

## Schizophrenia Studies

In a National Institute of Mental Health study involving schizophrenic patients treated for 2 years with either exploratory, insight-oriented psychotherapy three times a week or the control therapy (called reality-adaptive, supportive psychotherapy) once a week, there was clear evidence of a better outcome for patients treated with the supportive psychotherapy (Gunderson et al. 1984; Stanton et al. 1984). All patients were maintained on their usual medications throughout the study.

In another study, schizophrenic patients were randomly assigned to supportive therapy or family treatment (Rea et al. 1991). Patients were treated for 9 months and followed for 2 years. Supportive therapy consisted of medication case management, crisis intervention, and education about schizophrenia, whereas family treatment involved problem-solving therapy and communication-skills training. Patients in supportive treatment had significant improvement in coping style compared with patients in family therapy. However, the two treatment groups were not at comparable levels of coping skills, and this fact was not considered in the statistical analysis.

Hogarty et al. (1997) stated that supportive psychotherapy fares less well compared with other psychosocial approaches, such as family psychoeducation, skills training, or role therapy. However, defining *supportive therapy* as not including psychoeducation, skills training, or role therapy approaches is problematic because most therapists practicing supportive psychotherapy commonly employ these approaches. More recent psychotherapy approaches with schizophrenic patients include social skills training, which may be enhanced with amplified skills training in the community (Glynn et al. 2002; Liberman et al. 1998).

## Depressive Disorder Studies

In the National Institute of Mental Health Treatment of Depression Collaborative Research Program, two psychotherapies (cognitive-behavioral therapy and interpersonal therapy) were compared with an antidepressant (imipramine)–clinical management condition and a control condition consisting of drug placebo and clinical management (Elkin 1994; Elkin et al. 1989; Imber et al. 1990). The clinical management was a low-level supportive therapy approach. The two psychotherapies were found to be efficacious but not significantly different from the placebo–clinical management condition on measures of depressive symptoms and overall functioning.

Thompson and Gallagher (1985) studied 30 outpatients ranging in age from 60 to 81 years. Patients were randomly assigned to a 16-week treatment with cognitive therapy, behavior treatment, or supportive psychotherapy. Improvement was similar across the three treatment conditions at termination, but at 1-year follow-up, more of the patients in supportive therapy received a diagnosis of depression. Unfortunately, the small number of patients in each treatment group, as well as the type of supportive therapy used, makes these findings of limited value.

In a randomized clinical trial involving 100 depressed adolescents, Renaud et al. (1998) compared cognitive, family, and supportive psychotherapies and found that rapid responders to therapy had better outcomes at 1-year follow-up and better scores on some measures at 2-year follow-up. The investigators concluded that their findings suggest that patients with milder forms of depression may benefit from initial supportive psychotherapy or short trials of more specialized types of psychotherapy.

## Anxiety Disorder Studies

Systematic hierarchical desensitization was compared with supportive psychotherapy in a 26-week treatment trial involving patients with various types of phobias (Klein et al. 1983). Both treatments performed well, and there was no difference between the two approaches. The authors speculated that for phobic individuals, psychotherapy serves as an instigator of corrective activity outside the formal session by maintaining exposure in vivo. In another study, patients with phobias and panic attacks received either imipramine plus behavior therapy or imipramine plus supportive psychotherapy (Zitrin et al. 1978). The majority of patients showed moderate to marked improvement, and there was no difference between behavior therapy and supportive therapy in terms of improvement rates. In a study of social anxiety (phobia), Alstrom and colleagues (1984) found that supportive psychotherapy and prolonged exposure therapy were equally effective. However, Shear et al. (2001) reported that emotion-focused psychotherapy, a form of supportive therapy, has low efficacy for the treatment of panic disorder. They compared emotion-focused psychotherapy with cognitive-behavioral treatment, imipramine, or pill placebo in a study involving 112 subjects.

## Personality Disorder Studies

In a study comparing supportive with interpretive psychotherapy, Piper and colleagues (1998) found no outcome differences between the two treatments. Patients presented with anxiety or depressive disorders, and 60.4% of subjects had comorbid personality disorder. Another study involving personality disorder patients, comparing brief supportive therapy with short-term dynamic psychotherapy, found similar efficacy on measures of symptomatology, presenting complaints, and interpersonal functioning (Hellerstein et al. 1998). Patients had primarily Cluster C and "not otherwise specified" personality disorders, as well as comorbid Axis I disorders, such as depression or anxiety. These changes were found not only at termination but also at 6-month follow-up. In a substudy of the study by Hellerstein and colleagues (1998), the authors used the Inventory of Interpersonal Problems mapped to an interpersonal circumplex model and graphically demonstrated lasting positive change in interpersonal functioning in subjects treated with supportive psychotherapy (Rosenthal et al. 1999; Winston et al. 2001).

## Medical Disorder Studies

Mumford et al. (1982) reviewed controlled studies of supportive psychotherapy—including education about illness and treatments, cognitive-behavioral techniques, and ventilation and reassurance in a supportive relationship—in patients recovering from myocardial infarctions and surgery. The authors found better experiences with pain and increased patient compliance and speed of recovery, as well as fewer complications and fewer days in the hospital.

## Conclusion

This brief review of the efficacy of supportive psychotherapy indicates that supportive treatment appears to be useful across a broad spectrum of psychiatric and medical disorders. However, more research is needed to clarify the indications for supportive psychotherapy and how this treatment should be integrated with other psychotherapy approaches and treatment with medication.

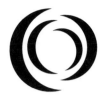

# 5

# General Framework of Supportive Psychotherapy

## Indications and Contraindications

Supportive psychotherapy was described for years as the treatment for individuals not suitable for expressive therapies—persons who are difficult to treat or for whom expressive techniques are expected to fail (Rosenthal et al. 1999; Winston et al. 1986). From this perspective, supportive psychotherapy was said to be indicated for people who have 1) a predominance of primitive defenses (e.g., projection and denial); 2) an absence of capacity for mutuality and reciprocity, exemplifying an impairment in object relations; 3) an inability to introspect; 4) an inability to recognize the object as separate from the self, because of malignant narcissism or autism; 5) inadequate affect regulation, especially in the form of aggression; 6) somatoform problems; and 7) overwhelming anxiety related to issues of separation or individuation (Buckley 1986; Werman 1984).

However, the findings of the Menninger psychotherapy study indicated that patients treated with supportive psychotherapy made greater-than-expected gains (compared with patients who received psychoanalytic treatments) and may have achieved lasting character change (Wallerstein 1989). In addition, data from recent research support the premise that higher-functioning patients for whom expressive treatments have traditionally been indicated respond just as well to supportive treatment, in terms of reduction of target complaints and psychiatric symptoms (Hellerstein et al. 1998), and develop a more differentiated and adaptive self because of the interactions in supportive psychotherapy. These changes can be measured as lasting reductions in intensity of patient-rated interpersonal problems after termination of treatment (Rosenthal et al. 1999).

These findings suggest not only that supportive psychotherapy is broadly applicable, including in areas where traditional expressive treatments are not indicated, but also that it can be used successfully with a wide spectrum of problems and with higher-functioning patients. Indeed, the most widely used form of psychotherapy is supportive psychotherapy with some expressive elements. Luborsky (1984) and others developed various forms of supportive-expressive psychotherapy that have produced positive results in clinical trials. Supportive psychotherapy is the probably the best initial approach when psychotherapeutic intervention is being considered (Hellerstein et al. 1994). The therapist should move away from supportive psychotherapy only when there is a positive indication for another specific treatment. In addition to the use of supportive psychotherapy as a starting point in the decision tree for differential psychotherapeutics, there are several indications for which supportive psychotherapy has the best contextual fit and specific efficacy. The indications are discussed in detail in Chapter 8, "Applicability to Special Populations."

## Indications

Indications for supportive psychotherapy reiterated in the older literature are essentially a statement of contraindications for treatment at the most expressive pole of the supportive-expressive continuum. These indications for supportive psychotherapy conceptually fall into two groups, which are not really discrete: 1) crisis, which includes acute illnesses that emerge with the overwhelming of the patient's defenses in the context of intense physical or psychological stress; and 2) chronic illness with concomitant impairment of adaptive skills and psychological functions.

### Crisis

Persons in whom crisis is an indication for supportive psychotherapy are relatively well-functioning and well-adapted individuals who have become symptomatic in the context of acute, overwhelming, or unusual stress. In other circumstances, persons in this group might be referred for expressive treatment, because these individuals have good reality testing, a capacity to tolerate and contain affects and impulses, good object relations, a capacity to form a working alliance, and some capacity for introspection.

In the case of this group, supportive psychotherapy is usually delivered in an acute-care or episodes-of-care model. For example, an otherwise well-compensated patient having a strong depressive reaction to the change in her body image after a mastectomy, with accompanying loss of self-esteem and a negative attitude toward work and social relationships, may be able to make use of the psychological support of and empathic interaction with a therapist until she begins to grieve what has been lost, begins to master the situation, revises her expectations and plans, and renormalizes her daily life.

Following are some of the diagnostic and situational indications that fall into the category of crisis.

**Acute crisis.** Acute crisis is not a diagnosis but rather a general syndromal description for patients whose customary coping skills and defensive maneuvers have been overwhelmed by an (often unexpected) event, resulting in intense anxiety and other symptoms (Dewald 1994). Crisis is the state that people experience when they are faced with actual, impending, or possible loss: loss of life from a life-threatening illness, loss of liberty for a criminal offense, loss of personal or public safety (e.g., after the terrorist attacks of September 11, 2001, on New York and Washington, DC), or loss of a loved one. (See Chapter 7, "Crisis Intervention," for a more complete discussion.) Supportive techniques may even be implemented in the middle of expressive therapies when there is a crisis for which support is clinically indicated.

**Adjustment disorders, in relatively well-compensated people.** People in crisis may meet criteria for an adjustment disorder. Adjustment disorders are self-limited, lasting no more than 6 months (American Psychiatric Association 2000), and supportive psychotherapy can at least help the patient to manage uncomfortable feeling states and to shore up or develop coping strategies while the patient and therapist wait for the episode to end. The focus of the treatment is 1) to reassure the patient that symptoms are time limited, 2) to reduce stress by clarifying and providing information about that which the patient is having difficulty adjusting to, and 3) to support novel coping and problem-solving methods, including environmental change (Misch 2000). At its best, supportive psychotherapy facilitates a more rapid diminution in symptoms and resolution of the episode, and the treatment might help prevent the condition from becoming chronic.

**Medical illness.** For a large number of medical conditions, supportive psychotherapy is the only treatment recommended. An understanding of the individual's innate defensive, cognitive, and interpersonal styles (i.e., the core character and personality) enables the therapist to assist the patient in developing better coping strategies (Bronheim et al. 1998).

Supportive or supportive-expressive psychotherapy has been recommended for or has shown utility in reducing pain intensity and interference with normal work, sleep, and enjoyment of life in patients with HIV-related neuropathic pain (Evans et al. 2003); reducing the frequency and impact of stressful events in patients with primary (Hunter et al. 1996) or metastatic (Classen et al. 2001) breast cancer; treating HIV-positive patients with depression (Markowitz et al. 1995); treating patients with pancreatic cancer (Alter 1996); treating cancer patients with depression (Massie and Holland 1990) or chronic pain (Thomas and Weiss 2000); and treating hospitalized patients with somatization disorder (Quality Assurance Project 1985).

**Substance use disorders.** Early in the treatment of substance dependence, the therapist focuses on development of a therapeutic alliance, to assist treatment retention and to create a context within which the patient can begin cognitive and motivational work to assist recovery efforts (O'Malley et al. 1992). Kaufman and Reoux (1988) suggested that in the case of patients with substance dependence, expressive therapies (when appropriate) should not commence until the patient has implemented a concrete method of maintaining sobriety, because expressive therapies provoke anxiety that may trigger relapse. (A broader discussion of substance use disorders is found in Chapter 8, "Applicability to Special Populations.")

**Acute bereavement.** Acute bereavement in patients with poor ego strength will overwhelm their coping skills and defensive operations, producing symptoms such as self-reproach, social withdrawal, an inability to process the object loss, anxiety and depressive symptoms such as insomnia and anorexia, and an inability to maintain job or interpersonal functioning (Horowitz et al. 1984). Supportive psychotherapy affords the patient an empathic holding environment wherein he or she can talk and ventilate about both pain and hostility, have his or her self-esteem directly supported through reassurance and appropriate praise, gain direction for activities of daily living, and reality-test his or her role in the deceased's life and death. The process supports the use of healthy defensive operations, concrete assistance for routine activities the patient is not able to perform, and appropriate reaching out as a measure against the tendency to remain socially withdrawn (Novalis et al. 1993).

**Alexithymia.** Patients who are typically characterized as alexithymic demonstrate characteristics that make expressive therapy difficult if not impossible. These characteristics include severe restriction of affect, a seeming lack of capacity for introspection, an inability to articulate feeling states, and a diminished or absent fantasy life (Sifneos 1973, 1975). When these patients become symptomatic because of stressors such as acute medical illness, they may become somatically preoccupied and increasingly dysfunctional, but they are still unable to communicate the effect of the stress on their affective experience. Supportive psychotherapy, through working directly on somatic experiences and personal metaphors, can specifically address alexithymia in helping the patient to recognize, acknowledge, identify, and label emotions and thus increase a sense of mastery and self-esteem (Misch 2000).

### Chronic Illness

Compared with individuals in crisis, individuals who must cope with chronic mental illness are more traditionally associated with supportive psychotherapy and are more likely to entail longer-term therapy (Drake and Sederer 1986; Kates and Rockland 1994; Werman 1984). Patients in this category typically have a decrease in self-esteem related to deficits in adaptive skills and ego functioning. This group not only includes patients with Axis I disorders that have a chronic or intermittent course, but also typically includes patients who have moderate to severe personality disorders and whose idiosyncratic interpersonal style, adaptive skills, and ego deficits are chronic, pervasive, and maladaptive (Sampson and Weiss 1986). The majority of psychotherapy patients in outpatient psychiatric clinics have probably been treated with dynamically informed supportive psychotherapy.

Some chronic conditions not usually associated with severe mental illness can be damaging to adaptive and psychological functioning and may be positively affected by supportive psychotherapy. These conditions include later stages of severe medical illness, when the patient is not expected to recover but when supportive psychotherapy can be expected to assist the patient in reducing suffering and in maintaining self-esteem, adaptive skills, and ego functioning for as long as practicable (Thomas and Weiss 2000).

## Contraindications

Because supportive psychotherapy is based on the factors common to all psychotherapies, there are relatively few circumstances in which it is contraindicated (Frank 1975; Pinsker et al. 1996). We have argued that supportive psychotherapy is the appropriate default approach to psychotherapy (Hellerstein et al. 1994) and that supportive psychotherapy thus can be applied over a wide range of psychopathology and situations. Put more plainly, supportive psychotherapy is contraindicated when psychotherapy itself is contraindicated. Fortunately, the list of contraindications is a short one.

Novalis et al. (1993) suggested that supportive psychotherapy is unlikely to be effective in delirium states, other organic mental disorders, drug intoxication, and later stages of dementia, but these are conditions in which any psychotherapy could be expected to fail. Help-rejecting complainers, because they are wedded to the victim role and are not invested in becoming more adaptive, do not make good use of supportive interventions but rather become worse as they confirm that the goodwill and concrete advice of the therapist are not useful. Con artists and others who lie or malinger as a matter of course do as poorly in this treatment as in other treatments. Psychopathic individuals, who establish a pattern of pseudomutuality in the therapeutic relationship, either quickly understand the lack of opportunity for real gratification and so drop out of treatment, or become focused on attempting to use the relationship to inappropriately gratify real or imagined needs. In the latter case, the therapist experiences the patient as being increasingly needy in order to elicit the therapist's goodwill and expected concrete gain, or the patient becomes coercive to achieve the same goals.

The contraindications for supportive psychotherapy are few. A more formal cognitive-behavioral treatment appears to be more effective than supportive psychotherapy for some conditions, including Tourette's disorder (Wilhelm et al. 2003); acute adolescent depression (Brent et al. 1997), although cognitive-behavioral therapy does not have a better effect on long-term outcome (Birmaher et al. 2000); panic disorder (Beck et al. 1992); obsessive-compulsive disorder (Foa and Franklin 2002); and bulimia nervosa (Walsh et al. 1997). The integration of supportive psychotherapy and cognitive-behavioral therapy was discussed at length by Winston and Winston (2002).

# Initiation of Treatment

If the therapist determines that supportive psychotherapy is the treatment of choice, he or she will make that determination during the first session, and thus the therapist will essentially be conducting supportive psychotherapy in the first session (see Chapter 4, "Assessment, Case Formulation, Goal Setting, and Outcome Research"). Therefore, history taking, payment negotiations, interchanges on the rules and conduct of therapy, goal setting, and length-of-treatment discussions are conducted much as in the rest of the treatment. Supportive psychotherapy, which is conversational in style and serves as the context for all patient–therapist interactions, has no artificial boundary and thus is "always on."

During the initial sessions, the ground rules of supportive psychotherapy should be made explicit. It is important to obtain the patient's agreement about these ground rules. The therapist may need to temper the message, depending on the characteristics of the patient—including educational level, ego strength, reality testing, and context of treatment—but the overall idea in creating an unambiguous format for the rules of engagement in therapy is to reduce anxiety by setting clear limits. The most obvious general rules are the following: 1) in the session, there will be no physical aggression and no verbal abuse; and 2) patients should not come for treatment in an intoxicated state.

## Office Arrangement

### Seating

Seating for supportive psychotherapy is best arranged in a manner that is welcoming, friendly, comfortable, and professional—just like the treatment itself. Thus, one should provide adequate but not harsh lighting, and comfortable chairs that are not too close but also not too far away, so that participants can sit upright and see and hear each other easily. The therapist can then pick up nuances of verbal tone, facial expression, and body language. Doing so is important because supportive psychotherapy is dynamic in its understanding. The therapist is sensitive to unconscious communication, even if he or she does not make that awareness explicit to the patient in the form of confrontation or interpretation. Physical distance is flexible in response to clinical need. The therapist may sit a little farther away than usual when respecting the need for distance in a patient who expresses paranoid ideation. Conversely, when the therapist is too far away, the patient's anxiety may increase, because talking face-to-face with someone for an extended length of time from 10 feet away is socially unusual. There may be times when the patient–therapist proximity is closer than usual (e.g., when the therapist is conducting supportive psychotherapy by sitting next to a patient who is confined to a hospital bed).

## Amenities

In the past, the literature about supportive psychotherapy framed the therapy as a treatment for the most impaired, unpsychologically minded individuals. In this vein, it was suggested that—in contrast to the abstaining, nongratifying position of the therapist in expressive treatments—the supportive psychotherapist provide, in his or her office, small comforts to the patient in the form of a box of facial tissues on the table and a small plate of cookies or other treats by the door. All psychotherapy should be provided in a humane and respectful fashion in a reasonable setting, and we suggest that this aim can generally be achieved without resorting to feeding the patient in order to supply a positive image of the therapist. However, with the most impaired patients, provision of practical items (such as transportation tokens) and snacks likely help to sustain the therapeutic alliance. Feeding a patient is concretely accommodating him or her and providing a supportive relationship but is typically a part of supportive psychotherapy with the lowest-functioning patients. Similarly, gifts from the therapist to the patient are not expressly prohibited if the gift is related to the therapy, such as an informational manual, or if an institutional practice has been developed to supply items of need to the most needy patients (Novalis et al. 1993).

# Initiation and Termination of Sessions

The therapist is expected to begin and end sessions on time. This temporal framing of sessions is out of respect both for the patient and for the psychotherapist. Occasional lateness is not a typical issue to be focused on in supportive psychotherapy. When a patient demonstrates a pattern of lateness, the pattern can be explored within the supportive framework. In expressive treatment, the therapist labels the pattern of lateness and adheres to the assumption that the lateness is due to resistance or other unconscious processes. He or she then encourages the patient's verbalization, with the objective of maximizing the transference process. In supportive psychotherapy, the therapist is free to discuss matters of lateness from a practical point of view. Keeping appointments is adaptive behavior; coming late to a meeting that is genuinely in the patient's best interests is not. Such lateness can be attended to using a collaborative, problem-solving approach. A pattern of missing sessions can be addressed in the same way.

Here, the therapist discusses the patient's lateness:

Patient: Sorry, I'm late again. I just don't know—I was sure I gave myself
    enough time. [*angry*] No matter how I try, I'm always late to every-

thing! I do everything wrong! I should just go home! (***Overinclu-sive negativism, nihilism, defeatism***)

Therapist: I know it can feel that way, because it's frustrating to have a habit that gets in the way, but bad habits can be broken. [*engaging smile*] Are you sure you do *everything* wrong? If that were the case, you wouldn't have made it here at all today, and if you did get here, you might have forgotten your socks! (***Slogans, humor; challenges the negative self-statements***)

Patient: Okay, okay, maybe not everything! [*begrudging smile*] I just hate it when I'm late! It feels like someone's got a fix in against me, no matter how hard I try. (***Esteem-lowering experience of powerlessness, and projection***)

Therapist: That sure can't make you feel good about yourself. Can we look perhaps at how you decide what time to leave? Sometimes if people anticipate things happening, there's some wiggle room that will be taken up by unforeseen events and leave you enough time to get to an appointment. That would increase your sense of control over things and make you feel better. Want to give it a shot? (***Empathy and anticipatory guidance***)

Patient: Sure.

Similarly, a patient may establish a pattern of not stopping at the appropriate time, which might have different unconscious motivations, all amenable to discussion in the context of supporting ego function and adaptive skills. With some patients and in certain cases, it may be therapeutically appropriate to extend the time of a session. For example, when the patient is unavoidably detained by traffic but is in a crisis, the therapist may choose to give some extra time if his or her schedule allows, or may take the time to briefly connect and reschedule the next appointment if an earlier time is available. Similarly, when patients bring up what Pinsker (1997) called "doorknob issues"—issues brought up as the patient is exiting the session—the therapist is clinically compelled to take some extra minutes to address clinically provocative communications that raise acute concern in the therapist. Concerns about not gratifying the patient's infantile wishes should be entertained but should take a second place to reasonableness, which is the therapist modeling behavior.

However, the therapist may determine at times not to extend a session, because to do so would support maladaptive, regressive behavior without reasonable clinical or environmental justification. Thus, choosing not to extend a session is also modeling behavior for the patient. The therapist must balance limit setting with promotion of autonomy and independence, part of what Misch (2000) called "being a good parent" in supportive psychotherapy (see Chapter 1, "Basic Principles of Supportive Psychotherapy"). Sometimes, such promotion means getting up, opening the door, and firmly showing the patient out. Also, the therapist who recognizes that his or her patient continually resists the therapist's efforts to stop on time can choose to cue the patient at intervals about how much time is remaining in the session, thus offering anticipatory guidance. The experienced therapist uses these strategies to wind down a session before time is up, so that patients are not in the middle of a hot topic at the session's end (Pinsker 1997).

# Timing and Intensity of Treatment

The timing and intensity of treatment should be set through agreement of the patient and therapist, with the proviso that these aspects may change on the basis of clinical need—for example, when a crisis arises. Expressive treatments attempt to meet an ideal of a constant interval and time, but in supportive psychotherapy, the frequency of visits is less fixed. However, setting a specific, repeated time to meet tends to reduce anxiety, which is an intention of supportive treatment. Similarly, the length of a session should generally be fixed but be subject to variation when clinically appropriate and when the therapist can accommodate.

## Phases of Treatment

### Beginning

During the beginning of therapy, the therapist pays specific attention to supporting the formation of a therapeutic alliance, because such an alliance increases the likelihood that the patient will remain in treatment and will have a good outcome (Gunderson et al. 1984; Hartley and Strupp 1983). Over the first few sessions, the therapist should attempt to come to a reasonable understanding of the patient's target complaints and presenting symptoms and to acquire a working knowledge of the patient's general level of ego function and object relatedness, as well as his or her adaptive strengths and deficits. From these data, the therapist synthesizes a case formulation and hypothesizes areas of acute and chronic deficit in defensive operations, adaptive skills, and ego functioning that supportive interventions should directly address. As the therapist gets to know the patient better, the therapist will fine-tune his or her understanding of the patient's ego functioning and adjust the intensity of supportive and expressive interventions accordingly. It may take an extended time for the therapist to develop a clear understanding of the issues with patients who are cognitively impaired because of psychosis, severe obsessive thinking, or mood disorder, or with patients who become flooded with anxiety or dysphoria when certain details are focused on.

Once the goals and objectives of therapy are agreed on (see Chapter 4, "Assessment, Case Formulation, Goal Setting, and Outcome Research"), the therapist must consider issues of acuity and timing. For example, after a recent psychiatric hospitalization for psychosis, a patient comes in with the agenda of wanting to talk about whether he should reregister for classes in the fall. The therapist's clinical understanding is that the patient must secure a stable and structured environment to live in so that he can plan his near-term future appropriately. Without that stability, the patient runs the near-term risk of increased stress, disorganization, and decompensation. However, the patient has brought up neither the imminent loss of his housing nor his plans to deal with that loss. The therapist understands, before the patient does, the need to address certain issues or to address issues in a different order.

The therapist allows the patient to see the map before exploring the territory, an important supportive approach that reduces anxiety and emphasizes that therapy is a rational and collaborative process (Rosenthal 2002). The therapist can explain how the topic about to be discussed is specifically connected to self-esteem, to a specified ego function, or to a specified adaptive skill for dealing with psychiatric symptoms or general social interaction. Such explanation is also consistent with motivational interviewing approaches, in that the therapist asks the patient's permission before giving direct advice or prescribing solutions to problems (Rollnick and Miller 1995). However, the therapist must accept that at times, the patient will reject the proposed agenda.

## Middle Stages

Supportive psychotherapy is a therapy in which the therapeutic alliance probably functions as a foundation for treatment rather than as the vehicle for change (Hellerstein et al. 1998). Therefore, the therapist continues to monitor the alliance with the patient during the course of treatment and attempts to optimize that alliance using the same attention he or she used in the initial sessions of the treatment. This type of therapeutic attunement to the patient contributes to the patient's experience of being understood and supported by the therapist. In the middle phase of therapy, if therapy is proceeding well, the patient begins to accept that the therapist is truly capable of understanding and supporting him or her, and this acceptance can serve as a corrective emotional experience. Positive transference and regard for the therapist are allowed to accumulate in the therapist's account without interpretation, unless grossly pathological. In supportive treatment, the middle stage can and often does go on indefinitely, especially with patients for whom support helps to maintain adaptive skills or ego functions. During the course of treatment, new, intermediate goals may arise for the patient in the context of life events or increases in adaptive function. An increase in adaptive function presents an opportunity to review goals and to offer praise for meeting goals—and an opportunity to offer reassurance and other support for self-esteem with regard to goals that have not been accomplished.

On the platform of supportive psychotherapy, the therapist has room to use well-structured pychoeducational and skills-building interventions, as well as patient-driven processes or initiatives. At times during the course of treatment, the therapist can bring in expert knowledge to inform the patient about his or her disorder and its effect on functioning and to increase awareness so that the patient's decisions are better informed. With addicted patients, these kinds of educational interventions happen early and frequently in supportive psychotherapy and may increase motivation for behavioral change. At other times, the patient may come in with a pressing agenda in relation to an acute interpersonal circumstance, such as a dispute with a colleague at work. The supportive therapist will be able to shift the balance from therapist-directed to patient-directed processes, keeping both the patient's goals and the therapist's objectives in mind.

## Termination

A formal termination process is not part of supportive psychotherapy. Therapy ends when the goals of treatment have been reached or when the patient elects not to continue. If the therapist believes that the decision to stop is a product of ego function disturbance (e.g., grandiosity), symptoms (e.g., hopelessness), or faulty adaptive skills (e.g., inability to manage regular visits), the therapist attempts, without arguing, to explore the problem. Even when the therapist has a psychodynamic hypothesis about the patient's motivation, this hypothesis must be balanced against the proposition, fundamental to supportive psychotherapy, that the patient is free to stop when he or she wishes. Therapy may also terminate because of external factors such as relocation or another life event that forces an end to the current scope of work.

At the end of formal treatment, gains are summarized and an agenda is articulated for the patient's continued work without regular visits to the therapist. It is important for the patient to reflect on and celebrate important milestones that he or she has been able to achieve (Rosenthal 2002).

Supportive psychotherapy differs from expressive treatment with regard to termination in that the relationship with the therapist is not worked through with the intent of getting the patient to mourn the loss of an important object and to work through ambivalent feelings (Rosenthal 2002). Because constant, positively held objects are frequently too few in the lives of many of these patients, supportive psychotherapy does not attempt to get the patient to let go of the relationship with the therapist, which is based in the real relationship rather than in the transference. The analogy of school is useful. The teacher works in the school even when the student is not enrolled in classes. Treatment can be framed as an organized set of courses, each with a beginning, middle, and end. When the achievement of goals are met, the course of treatment is concluded. The student who has a worthwhile experience may return for more schooling (Pinsker and Rosenthal 1988). The patient is always told that he or she should feel free to come back should the need arise.

## Long-Term Versus Brief Therapy

For patients with chronic mental disorders, for whom supportive psychotherapy is mostly aimed at maintaining adaptive and ego functioning, treatment is likely to be framed as an ongoing relationship without a time limit, unless constrained by external factors, such as the patient's financial resources, insurance coverage, or continued-stay criteria in a mental health clinic. At the same time, treatment does not need to go on interminably, if the goals have been met.

Brief therapy is typically indicated when the psychopathology is expected to be time limited, such as in an adjustment disorder, in a terminal illness, or when an acute loss or a crisis overwhelms a patient's defenses and he or she becomes symptomatic. Because the model of treatment does not focus on character change through emotional insight, treatment is complete not when core conflicts have been resolved but rather when symptoms have been reduced to comfortable levels or when more-competent coping strategies have been developed. A patient may return for more treatment when in a crisis, or if there is again need to shore up failing defensive operations, or if the patient wants to work on something new.

## **Professional Boundaries**

Although it is never the therapist's turn—that is, the dialogue is always focused with the patient's therapeutic needs in mind—the style is conversational, to reduce awkward, anxiety-provoking silences. The therapist's empathic relatedness allows him or her to know both when silence will make the patient withdraw and feel overwhelmed and when it's time to be quiet and allow the patient to manifest an important affective response:

Patient 1 [*after a long pause, a tentative smile*]: Boy, it's been raining non-stop for so long.

Therapist 1: Sure has! Isn't it interesting? Folks often chat about the weather when they're not sure what else they have in common to talk about. It's kind of neat—there's always going to be weather! I wonder if you'd like to talk about how all that rain has affected you, but we can also discuss strategies to talk with people; you told me that's been a problem. (**Normalizing, generalizing, collaborating, anticipatory guidance**)

Patient 2 [*after a long pause, tears well up*]: I can't believe she's really gone.
Therapist 2: [*silent*] (**Attentive, quiet; empathic concern**)

In expressive treatment, in order to prevent gratification of the patient's wishes and to promote elaboration of transference material, self-disclosure of any sort is typically avoided. In supportive psychotherapy, the therapist may judiciously disclose personal information to the patient in a purposeful and supportive manner. The paradigmatic model of therapeutic self-disclosure is found in Alcoholics Anonymous and other self-help groups. A speaker's lived experience becomes an object lesson for listeners seeking support for their recovery efforts. Many reports on individual behavioral, cognitive, and cognitive-behavioral therapies suggest that deliberate self-disclosure can be clinically useful (Psychopathology Committee of the Group for the Advancement of Psychiatry 2001). Simon (1988) observed that therapists' decisions about deliberate self-disclosure are generally related to several criteria: modeling and educating, promoting the therapeutic alliance, validating reality, and fostering the patient's sense of autonomy. As a rule, self-disclosure by the therapist is appropriate when it is in the interest of the patient's treatment. If self-disclosure is in the therapist's interest (e.g., when it takes the form of ventilating, bragging, complaining, or seductiveness), it is exploitation. Information that is a matter of public record is typically the easiest to reveal in the context of supportive treatment. More private information or personal experience requires more deliberation. In supportive psychotherapy, the therapist looks for ways to add facilitating comments or interjections that normalize the interaction and to respond to inquiries in a manner that is both appropriate and technically supportive:

Patient [*after a long pause*]: I was thinking, are you married?
Therapist 1 [*if the therapist chooses to answer*]: What are your thoughts about this? (**Expressive-style response**)

Therapist 2: Yes, I am. I noticed you seemed to think a while before you asked me. Was it a little uncomfortable to think of asking me that? (***Empathic concern***)

Patient [*short pause*] [*blushing*]: Yep…I thought it might be weird to ask.

Therapist 2: One of the rules here is that you get to speak your mind. It's good you were able to ask me, even though it made you uncomfortable. People who are able to master their fears tend to get more accomplished. (***Praise with modeling of adaptive behavior***)

At times, a patient will ask a question that is annoying or anxiety provoking to the therapist, one that is obviously inappropriate or extremely personal in nature:

Patient: I know you're married, but do you still masturbate?

Therapist 1: My sexual habits are personal, but we should talk about sexual issues if you are having concerns or problems about sex. (***Clearly reiterating a boundary rule and then offering the patient a chance to discuss sexual concerns***)

Patients with more severe disorders may have difficulty at times differentiating the friendly but professional relationship from friendship. The therapist clarifies and reinforces the boundaries in a nondemeaning way, without being evasive or insincere:

Patient: I've got some Aerosmith tickets! So, we could meet at the box office, and I could give you one. How about that?

Therapist: That's really kind of you. I know that the tickets are special to you, and I want you to understand that I really appreciate that you're thinking of me. It makes me think that our working together is valued by you. But for future reference, I'm not allowed to receive gifts of more than nominal value from my patients. Also, people who have given a lot of thought to these things have decided that it's probably best to keep therapy relationships separate from other kinds of relationships like friendships so that nothing interferes.

Patient: Ah, c'mon, doc—it's just a concert ticket! It would be fun.

Therapist 1: You know, I was never much into heavy metal music, didn't like it when I was younger, so I really wouldn't want to go now even if we knew each other under different circumstances. (***Responds truthfully but evasively***)

Therapist 2: I'd prefer to keep our time together focused on our work, which is about getting things done in a very special and professional way, not about friendship. I'm sorry if that's a disappointment. Can we talk about this some more? (***Takes responsibility for the therapeutic boundary but is real and empathic in the relationship***)

Because supportive psychotherapy is more verbally interactive than traditional expressive treatments, and because the therapist has more opportunity to be a real figure in relating to the patient, there is also more opportunity for flexibility in moving traditional boundaries. For example, in order to normalize when a patient is struggling with day-to-day functioning after losing a parent, the therapist may empathically disclose his or her own pain and loss of motivation when the therapist was in a state of grieving. However, with a less abstemious relationship, there is also more real opportunity for the therapist to use the therapy to gratify his or her own needs and violate the patient's boundaries. Although the repertoire of therapist behavior and speech is broader in supportive psychotherapy, there is a narrow but clear domain of unacceptable therapist behaviors that exploit patients: sexual contact, borrowing money, or accepting patient favors or information that benefits the therapist (e.g., stock tips, chores, or advice based on nonpublic information).

## Summary

Supportive psychotherapy is generally indicated as the starting place for a treatment relationship between a therapist and a patient and thus has few contraindications. Other forms of treatment are undertaken only if specifically indicated and only with the patient's agreement. The length and intensity of supportive treatment vary according to the patient's need and motivation, and termination does not require working through ambivalent feelings about the therapist. Treatment is focused on real relationships, including the patient's relationship with the therapist, but transference material should be discussed when indicated. Although supportive psychotherapy allows a broader range of supportive behaviors by the therapist compared with expressive treatment, supportive psychotherapy is still constrained by clear guidelines about permissible patient and therapist behavior in the treatment setting.

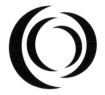

# 6

# The Therapeutic Relationship

**P**insker (1997) and others (Misch 2000; Novalis et al. 1993) described general principles of supportive psychotherapy that are related to the patient–therapist relationship. Some of these principles are listed here and are discussed further in the chapter.

1. Positive feelings toward and positive transferences to the therapist are generally not focused on in supportive psychotherapy, in order to sustain the therapeutic alliance.
2. The therapist is alert to distancing, negative responses in order to anticipate and avoid a disruption in treatment.
3. When a patient–therapist problem is not resolved through practical discussion, the therapist moves to discussion of the therapeutic relationship.
4. The therapist can modify the patient's distorted perceptions using clarification and confrontation and not interpretation.
5. If indirect means fail to address negative transference or therapeutic impasses, more explicit discussion about the relationship may be warranted.
6. The therapist uses only the amount of expressive technique necessary to address negative transference.
7. The therapeutic alliance may allow the patient to listen to the therapist present material that the patient would not accept from anyone else.

8. When making a statement that the patient will experience as criticism, sometimes the therapist will have to frame the statement in a palatable or supportive manner or first offer anticipatory guidance.

# Transference: Supportive and Expressive Approaches

*Transference* refers to the feelings, fantasies, beliefs, assumptions, and experiences concerning the therapist that do not originate in the therapist or in the patient's relationship with the therapist but rather are outgrowths from the patient's earlier relationships, unconsciously displaced on the therapist. Transference phenomena arise in all therapies, but the role assigned to transference in supportive psychotherapy is different from the role assigned to it in expressive psychotherapy.

In the most expressive psychotherapies and psychoanalysis—one pole of the expressive-supportive psychotherapy continuum described in Chapter 1, "Basic Principles of Supportive Psychotherapy"—transference phenomena are of pivotal importance for identifying intrapsychic conflicts; therapeutic gain is ascribed to the emotional working-through of these relationships. The patient–therapist relationship as expressed through transference phenomena is a major area of focus and engagement, whereas the working alliance or real relationship serves as a backdrop from which the patient's observing ego can peer onto the stage (Figure 6–1).

In psychotherapy at the supportive pole of the supportive-expressive psychotherapy continuum, transferences are recognized by the dynamically aware therapist and can be used to guide therapeutic interventions. However, transferences are not generally discussed, unless negative transference threatens to disrupt treatment. The real relationship between the patient and the therapist takes center stage (Figure 6–1).

However, between the two poles, where almost all psychotherapy takes place, a mixture of supportive and expressive approaches to transference material occurs. Supportive and expressive techniques can act as midwives to the emergence of the other at appropriate times in a treatment (Gorton 2000), but both the rationale for and content of transference interventions by the therapist are different in supportive and expressive treatments.

Supportive therapists track transference material but address it only when there is cause to do so. It is generally unnecessary to focus on positive transference material in supportive psychotherapy:

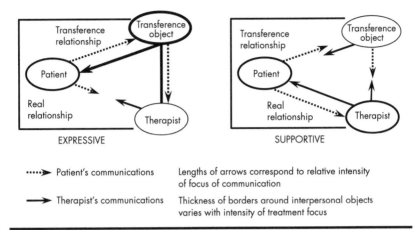

·····▷ Patient's communications   Lengths of arrows correspond to relative intensity
of focus of communication

──▶ Therapist's communications   Thickness of borders around interpersonal objects
varies with intensity of treatment focus

**Figure 6–1.**   Roles of transference and the real relationship in expressive and supportive psychotherapy.

*Source.*   Adapted from Pinsker et al. 1991.

> Patient: Doctor, you always give me the right advice, even when I'm not on the ball or I have some wrong idea. How'd you get so smart?
> Therapist: Thanks, Ben, but I can't take all the credit. I had good teachers, and I have learned a lot of effective principles from working with patients. (***Accepts the positive statement but modulates it slightly with reality testing***)

Negative transference is the phenomenon typically focused on in supportive psychotherapy, because such transference can be a threat to the integrity of the treatment and normally adds to the patient's suffering when acted on in the real world. In supportive and supportive-expressive psychotherapy, the therapist clarifies often, confronts at intervals, but interprets infrequently. The therapist's interventions assist the patient in recognizing and addressing maladaptive behavioral or construal patterns that are reflected in behavior with the therapist; a goal of these interventions is to increase self-esteem and adaptive functioning. The behavior with the therapist in supportive treatment is understood to be illustrative of the patient's behavior with others.

In expressive treatment, transference clarification and interpretation are important interventions. In this treatment, the patient's characterological and core neurotic defenses are often expressed through positive and negative transference phenomena. The therapist's transference interpretations and clarifications assist the patient in gaining insight and working through unconscious conflicts; a goal of these interventions is character change. In expressive therapy, relationships between the patient and other people are used to illuminate the central patient–therapist relationship.

The content of the therapist's transference interpretation also differs between expressive and supportive modes. The precision and comprehensiveness of an interpretation may vary, depending on the level of the patient's object relations and defensive functioning, the patient's progress in treatment, and the strength of the therapeutic alliance. Interventions often have more of the quality of clarifications and confrontations than interpretations in the strict sense. Typically, the healthier a patient is on the continuum of psychopathology, the better he or she will tolerate a precise and comprehensive interpretation without damaging the therapeutic alliance. However, interpretive ideas can be presented in a supportive manner (Winston et al. 1986). With more impaired patients, full interpretations are rarely made, but incomplete interpretations (leaving out genetic references and generalizing [Pinsker et al. 1991]) or inexact interpretations (diluting infantile fears with other plausible explanations [Glover 1931]) may be useful:

> Therapist 1: So keeping your room messy is a way for you to in a sense be independent and to do things in your own way in your own space, as compared with how it is at work, where everything must be annoyingly in its place and on time. Is there a downside? (*Supports self-esteem, makes a connection to angry feeling, contrasts patient's style with real-world expectation, opens a dialogue on adaptive skills*)

In the midst of an expressive treatment, the interpretation might be the following:

> Therapist 2: So keeping your room messy is a way of setting things up, hoping your mother cleans it up. She's supposed to make it OK, and you get anxious about it. Then you become enraged and feel you have little control. (*Makes a primary connection to a genetic figure and to the role of aggression in staving off anxiety when dependency needs are not met*)

## The Therapeutic Alliance

In supportive and supportive-expressive psychotherapies (e.g., brief supportive psychotherapy [Hellerstein et al. 1998], brief adaptive psychotherapy [Pollack et al. 1991], and supportive-expressive psychotherapy [Luborsky 1984]), an early and strong therapeutic alliance (which is reflective of the real relationship) is predictive of positive outcome in treatment and thus is a major focus of treatment (Westerman et al. 1995; Winston and Winston 2002).

In the early days of psychoanalysis, Freud acknowledged that transference included a personal relationship with the patient, which he called "rapport" or "unobjectionable positive transference." He considered this relationship necessary to maintain the motivation needed to collaborate effectively and therefore maintained that the relationship was not to be interpreted (Gill and Muslin 1976; Safran and Muran 2000). This view is the earliest evidence of a principle within psychodynamic treatments for managing a strong therapeutic alliance, and Freud's view lay the groundwork for the noninterpretation of positive transference in supportive psychotherapy. As the concept of the therapeutic alliance began to develop, the focus shifted to the working relationship between the patient and therapist and began to be framed as a "working alliance," with elements of the real relationship that were separate from the transference (Greenson 1965, 1967; Zetzel 1956).

Current conceptions of the alliance are broader and seem a commonsense fit with the construct of supportive psychotherapy. The strength of the therapeutic alliance hinges on the extent of agreement on therapeutic tasks and goals, the patient's capacity to perform the therapeutic work, the therapist's empathic relatedness and involvement, and the robustness of the affective bond between patient and therapist (Bordin 1979; Gaston 1990).

The therapeutic alliance is most likely the therapeutic foundation for change rather than the vehicle for change, as hypothesized for more expressive treatments (Gaston 1990; Hellerstein et al. 1998; Horvath and Symonds 1991). Therefore, the therapist fosters the alliance through active measures, acting as a good role model and "parent" and being tolerant and nonjudgmental (Misch 2000). Direct measures that support the self-esteem of the patient support the therapeutic alliance, which has a basis in the real relationship. The patient may have a fantasy about the therapist's capacities (transference), but the therapist is actively engaged with the patient in a real relationship and is providing help to the patient.

## Misalliance: Recognition and Repair

To promote effective psychotherapy, the therapist must pay attention to rifts in the alliance and make concerted efforts to repair them. In supportive treatment, because the therapist is active, there is more opportunity to say the wrong thing and to step on the patient's toes. However, there is also ample opportunity, as well as a breadth of strategy, in supportive treatment to intervene effectively in a rupture of the therapeutic alliance. Less constraint is placed on the ways in which the therapist might communicate to the patient his or her distress at being misunderstood, his or her sincere regret at having unwittingly impugned or patronized the patient, or his or her having raised a subject that the patient found intrusive, anxiety provoking, or simply unpalatable. Generally, when the therapist anticipates or notices a misalliance, he or she uses standard supportive techniques to address it, because supportive measures are the first line of repair for ruptures in the alliance (Bond et al. 1998). The therapist attempts to address the problem practically, in the context of the current situation, before moving to symbolic or transference issues (Pinsker 1997).

In the following example, the therapist deals with a rift in the therapeutic alliance:

Patient: I'm not sure why I'm here. [*sullen*]

Therapist: Could you clarify what you mean?

Patient: All we do is bicker back and forth, but he never owns up to anything. Just asks me questions, expects me to do what he wants, and never tells me what he really thinks. It's too much. I try to be reasonable, but it's always his way, and it's always my fault. Now it looks like it's over—the relationship's just over!

Therapist: I still don't understand. You've described this pattern here many times: having a good time followed by struggling with your boyfriend and thinking that it is over. But I'm unclear what you mean by your statement that you don't know why you're here. (*At-tempts, through clarification and confrontation, to get the patient to become more specific*)

Patient: What good is this? I talk and talk here, and another relationship is blowing up because I can't sustain it. I try to do the right thing, and it doesn't make any difference. I can't do it right enough. So I don't know what I'm doing here. (*Again, lodges a complaint about the treatment not giving her what she needs, despite her doing what she believes she is asked*)

Therapist: We look at the patterns in your relationship so that you can learn ways to change them or learn to do things in a different way, which can help your relationship and your self-esteem. (*Indirectly attempts to strengthen the therapeutic alliance by reiterating common goals*)

Patient: Ah, you're just like him! And I try to do it right, and it still doesn't work out. [*looks down, sullen*] (*Makes the attribution that the therapist behaves similarly to the patient's boyfriend, with similar effect*)

Therapist: I see. [*frowns*] I've been supporting you in working it out with him, "doing the right thing," but now you're stuck in this process that has you feeling one down, and not just with him, but here, too. And it's not working for you. (*"Owns up" to supporting the patient's staying in the relationship, which the patient feels diminishes her autonomy, because the relationship with the boyfriend reduces her self-esteem*)

Patient [*looks up at the therapist, alert*]

Therapist: In the past, I've supported your attempts to hold on to your relationship with this man, but you continue to have these powerful disputes where you end up feeling disempowered and blamed. While I can understand your disappointment and sadness about ending the relationship, I'm thinking that you are correct: trying to stay with him is too damaging to your self-esteem. Here I was trying to help you to stay and figure out a way to work it out, because I thought doing so was in your best interests, and now I think you know better about your own life. I'm sorry I didn't catch on earlier. Where do we go from here? *(At times, the therapist may have to change his or her position, as people normally do when talking with someone who is becoming angry or distant.)*

# Resistance

Many would say that the concept of resistance is relevant only to the expressive element of therapy, in which uncovering is essential. However, some use the term broadly to signify any patient-produced obstacle to achieving the goals of therapy. In this sense, we may characterize as resistance the nearly universal out-of-awareness fear of new ways and the tendency to cling to familiar patterns even when they are maladaptive. Because supportive treatment aims to support adaptive defenses and build self-esteem, the therapist's strategy in relation to resistance is to increase the patient's motivation for action through encouraging problem solving and the learning of new adaptive skills.

Another obstacle to treatment is a traitlike disposition to avoid painful affects, which can interfere even when the therapist makes every effort to mitigate discomfort or anxiety. In examining the traitlike components of resistance, Beutler and colleagues (2002b) presented evidence from several studies that measures of patient characteristics typically associated with trait resistance—such as defensiveness, anger, impulsivity, and direct avoidance—are negatively correlated with psychotherapy outcomes. These findings have direct relevance for supportive psychotherapy: patients with high levels of trait resistance tend to have better outcomes with dynamic nondirective, self-directed, or relationship-oriented therapies (e.g., supportive-expressive psychotherapies) than with structured cognitive or behavioral treatments (Beutler et al. 2002b).

## Supportive Techniques

### "Joining the Resistance"

Supportive treatment aims to support defenses unless they are maladaptive. Again, a primary principle in supportive psychotherapy is to support the therapeutic alliance. When a patient is resistant to looking at dysfunctional patterns, the fact that the therapist reflects the patient's despair and hopelessness or empathizes with his or her tough life or work situation might give the patient a strong sense of being understood and thus increase his or her willingness to work in therapy (Messer 2002). Supportive psychotherapy can provide, without coercion, an active empathic environment and reinforcement of the patient's stated goals.

In supportive-expressive treatment, when a patient is struggling with recognizing his or her own feelings or impulses, the therapist can follow the patient's lead and make empathic statements about how difficult and anxiety provoking it is to reveal oneself (Messer 2002):

> Patient: Mom was usually pretty good about getting to games on time, but Dad used to show up sometimes…usually after the fact.…He was always really busy…[*looks sad*] and we got along…OK [*pause*]. Hey, you know why I was late today? The cabdriver on the way here—the stupid guy couldn't drive worth a damn! What a joke. How'd he get a license?
>
> Therapist: It seems that it's making you anxious to focus on how you really feel toward your father.
>
> Patient: This is hard. I don't think I can do this. [*tearing*] What if I can't do this? (***Increased anxiety, self-doubt***)
>
> Therapist: Talking about this kind of difficult stuff makes people anxious, and they get through it in psychotherapy. I want you to know that your pursuing it and revealing it here takes courage. I think you're clearly capable of doing it. I wouldn't support your looking at it if I thought you weren't capable. (***Empathy, normalization, accurate praise, reassurance***)

## Reducing Anxiety to Facilitate Discussion

Showing the patient a map before exploring the territory reiterates that the engagement is collaborative and centers around agreed-on goals. Anxiety is often diminished when the patient becomes cognitively aware of what is being offered for discussion:

> Patient: Sorry I'm late. I started out with plenty of time, but some things came up, and before I knew it, it was 20 after.
>
> Therapist: Have you noticed that over the last few weeks, you've come into the session about 20 minutes before our time's up? I feel bad that you may not be getting what you are paying for. Could we talk about it? (***In another circumstance, the therapist might be unclear about whether consistent lateness is related to feelings about the therapy or the therapist or is due to deficits in ego function or adaptive skills. In this case, the therapist knows from earlier sessions that the patient's lateness is related to the therapist.***)

Patient: Sure, but I just had stuff to do, and I lost track of the time. (*Rationalizes, deflects, plays the lateness off as a result of making more important choices*)

Therapist: In psychotherapy, when someone creates a pattern of somehow getting to the session with only a little time left, it may mean that there is something the person is wrestling with inside that is showing up in this pattern, outside. People do well with looking at it, exploring it, though sometimes it brings up uncomfortable emotions. I'm happy to explore it with you if you are interested. It might be helpful. (*Clarifies, confronts, normalizes, offers guidance about the cost of exploring this issue*)

Patient: It's not just here, doc. I'm late for everything [*sheepish grin*]. (*Generalizes away from the therapy situation but owns the pattern*)

Therapist: So, as a bonus, if we can explore that pattern here, maybe you can learn a skill or a principle that helps you to get along better out there. Is that something you'd be interested in? (*Supports motivation, enlists collaboration*)

Patient: Sure.

## Reframing Resistance as Healthy Self-Assertion

The therapist can address opposition to his or her efforts by framing it as a healthy function of the patient's need for control and self-assertion; the therapist may reduce the resistance by becoming more accepting and authentic (Beutler et al. 2002a):

Patient: I didn't ask my mom to enroll me for the spring semester…like we talked about last time. I decided to put it off until the fall. I'm just not ready to do that yet. Are you angry?

Therapist: It's good that you know your own mind and can make a definitive decision. You must feel some relief about taking a stand. I'm not angry, because I don't get to make the decisions about your life, only to look at the decisions together with you and try to help you with how you make them.

## Dealing With Distance and Withdrawal

Patients frequently demonstrate resistance in session through withdrawal and noninteraction. Because verbal responsiveness on the part of the therapist is a characteristic of supportive psychotherapy, the therapist does not wait for things to unfold if the patient is silent. Doing so supports resistance and may increase the patient's anxiety. In supportive psychotherapy, when the patient is silent or unresponsive, the therapist selects an issue for attention. The issue may be directly related to the patient's lack of verbal engagement, which the therapist may choose to address indirectly—or not at all, by switching to another topic entirely:

Patient: Hello again. [*sits down*] I don't really have much to talk about to-day. [*sits quietly, looking at the therapist blankly*]

Therapist 1 [*warmly*]: It's good to see you again. So, can we get back to the topic you were discussing with me before I left on vacation? You were describing how hard it was to follow through on asking for a transfer at work and how those "Why bother?" thoughts were getting in your way. (*The therapist picks up the patient's topic from before the therapist's absence, reconnecting and supporting the patient's self-esteem by showing that the patient was important enough to the therapist for the therapist to remember the issue. This approach sidesteps what the therapist assumes are negative emotions about the therapist's absence and increased anxiety about revealing them, yet focuses indirectly on the patient's distancing maneuvers.*)

Therapist 2: Hello. It's good to see you again. Well, it's been 3 weeks since our last session. Although I had someone covering for emergencies, it's not the same as coming for therapy.

Patient: That's right. [*looks at the therapist less blankly*] (*Engages a bit, reinforces the therapist's coming in closer*)

Therapist 2: Sometimes, when people say they don't have anything on their mind or much to talk about, they actually do but aren't quite sure whether to or how to say something. Patients often find themselves in that situation when their therapists come back after a vacation. (*Clarifies the situation but generalizes away from the specifics of the patient and the therapist before confronting the patient's denial and withdrawal*)

The therapist must be alert to distancing, negative responses and be able to anticipate and avoid a disruption in treatment. Not addressing misalliance may lead to a treatment disruption. The therapist must decide whether it is necessary to intervene through confrontation or whether indirect means will suffice. The therapist must always evaluate, through introspection, and determine that he or she is not becoming involved in a countertransference enactment (Robbins 2000).

# Countertransference

"Asking patients to tell us what they want potentially opens an imagined Pandora's box of outrageous requests, and it requires energy both to negotiate this tactfully and to manage the countertransference such negotiation produces in ourselves" (Clever and Tulsky 2002, p. 893).

## Defining Countertransference

When we discuss countertransference, it is important to make a distinction between emotional reactions to a patient's behavior that are due to the therapist's issues, and emotional reactions that are the therapist's response to the patient's unconscious attempt to provoke a reaction, which might be a manifestation of transference, coming from the patient's internal world (Messer 2002). The first type of countertransference is what has been described as the narrow or classical view of countertransference, essentially the therapist's transference to the patient (Gabbard 2001). On a related note, when the therapist is lacking in expertise or when the type of therapy is not helpful for the patient or problem, the therapist may mistakenly identify his or her bad feelings about the patient and treatment as countertransference, or the therapist may misperceive the problem as the patient's resistance. The therapist makes an attribution that the patient is being resistant, but it is the therapist or treatment that is not effective.

Because we describe supportive psychotherapy as a dynamically informed treatment, the second or broader view of countertransference has a place in our discussion of technical work with patients. This view is that emotional reactions of the therapist to the patient represent useful information related to the patient's inner world and unconscious (Gabbard 2001). Currently, many psychoanalytic theorists from varying perspectives form a consensus view that countertransference is a transactional construct, affected by what the therapist brings to the situation as well as by what the patient projects (Gabbard 2001; Kiesler 2001). A discussion of therapist transference is beyond the scope of this chapter, but it is incumbent on the therapist to attempt to distinguish his or her own feelings from those provoked by the patient or, in the case of projective identification, those that arise in the patient.

Supportive psychotherapy aims to improve adaptive skills. Maladaptive behavior patterns in the patient's real life frequently present as countertransference elicitations in the therapy session. When the therapist recognizes that his or her reactions to the patient are the same as everyone else's reactions, sharing this awareness with the patient may be useful in framing practical interventions to assist the patient with better interpersonal adaptation. However, the therapist must be aware that his or her intent to self-disclose feelings toward the patient could represent the therapist's own needs, not the requirements of the therapeutic situation. Such an awareness is more important in supportive psychotherapy, in which the flow of dialogue is conversational, than in expressive treatment, in which the therapist relatively abstains from responding. Gelso and colleagues (1995, 2002) demonstrated that better countertransference management correlates positively with better outcome in brief therapy (12 sessions).

The therapist in the following dialogue recognizes the patient's maladaptive behavior pattern:

Patient: Everyone always blows me off. I try to be nice—you know…join in, tell stories and stuff—then I see them look at each other, and they throw it in my face, and they make excuses and leave. Like they're so cool. That Andy—he's a piece of work, and I told him so.

Therapist: It must be hard to try joining in and be rejected like that. (*Empathic*)

Patient: Stop talking down to me. Jeez, you shrinks always act like you're Mother Teresa, but she didn't take the money for herself, did she? (*Feels impugned, attacks by questioning the therapist's motives*)

Therapist: Hmm. It sounds like how you are being here with me is how you've described interacting with Andy and Fred at work. I'm finding my temperature rising with your criticisms of me, and I can't help but wonder if you get the guys at work to feel the same way—except I won't act on my feelings the way that they do. I'll continue to sit and talk with you; I won't make excuses and leave. (*Modulated confrontation, drawing of parallels. The therapist restates her commitment to the process and offers disconfirmation of the patient's expected rejection in spite of the pressure to reject the patient*)

Patient: Oh, sure! Now you're saying it's my fault you're angry? (*Continues the verbal assault, feels criticized anyway*)

Therapist: I think if we get into an argument, I won't be doing my job of being helpful to you, and you'll keep feeling put down. No, what I'm asking you to do is see if there is a pattern here that we can work on to help you to get along better with people, since you've told me you would like that. (*Clarifies, does not get pulled into acting out of countertransference feeling; recommits to the work, focuses on the alliance in spite of heightened feelings, reinforces the patient's treatment goal*)

From the vantage point of interpersonal communication theory, Kiesler (2001) described effective feedback of countertransference feelings as applying the principle that disclosing metaphors or fantasies has the least threatening effect, compared with direct feelings or tendencies toward action. This principle is highly consistent with supportive psychotherapy approaches, in which it is safer, more respectful, and more protective of the therapeutic alliance to say, "I'm finding my temperature rising" rather than "I'm so angry, I feel like punching you out." The therapist's modulated expression of countertransference feeling not only offers disconfirmation of the patient's maladaptive construal style but also models adult restraint and containment (but not denial) of affect. The therapist who responds to the patient's hostility in a complementarily hostile way is arguing. Besides being bad supportive technique, this type of response is predictive of poor outcome (Henry et al. 1986, 1990).

## Handling Devaluation

Being devalued by a patient can be a painful experience and is a frequent experience of therapists working with patients who have borderline or narcissistic psychopathology. The adaptive response of the therapist is to try to get the patient to understand the therapist's response as helpful and consistent with the goals of treatment rather than as retaliatory or as a way for the therapist to remove himself or herself as the object of the patient's aggression (Robbins 2000). The therapist must bind the affects and be aware of the countertransference responses elicited with the attack, including anger over the patient's display of narcissism:

> Patient: I needed that note from you, and you screwed up! I left word on your voice mail that I needed it by Monday. [*vindictive tone*] Figures, you could only get into medical school at a state school…
>
> Therapist 1 [*feels guilty*]: I'm really sorry. Next time I'll try to be more sensitive to your needs, but I was out on Monday. (**Masochistic countertransference response to what was actually an unreasonable demand, a mea culpa gratifying the patient's grandiose self**)
>
> Therapist 2 [*feels irritated*]: You're pretty quick to blame me and make critical comments, but you take no responsibility at all for what happened. You left the request over the weekend, and I was out on Monday. (**Accurate but critical rebuttal, which may leave the patient feeling demeaned and angry**)
>
> Patient: I've heard those excuses before! I needed you. Now, how can I *trust* you? I knew I should have gone to that Park Avenue shrink my mother told me about! He went to Harvard. He's quoted in the newspaper all the time.
>
> Therapist 3: Sometimes, I'm going to disappoint you. It happens, even in the best relationships. It might scare you or make you angry that I'm not perfectly attuned to your needs, but fortunately, I don't need to be perfect to be helpful to you. I'll bet that other psychiatrist doesn't need to be perfect either to be effective. (**Authentic but measured response. Models healthy, adult behavior that is neither retaliating nor capitulating; clarifies the role of a "good-enough" therapist**)

The therapist must have appropriate training and means to understand feelings of irritation, frustration, and helplessness generated in response to a patient's chronic criticism and devaluation. Without adequate peer support or professional supervision, the therapist may become clinically disenchanted or disempowered and become either bored or overly confrontational (Rosenthal 2002).

Distancing from empathic connection is a common therapist response to patients' projective identifications (Kaufman 1992). Rather than identifying with the patient's projections and either capitulating or counter-attacking, the therapist manages vulnerability and aggression in the context of being devalued. Such management is in concordance with supportive principles (Robbins 2000) and can allow the patient to establish an idealizing transference through which he or she can experience safety in relationship to the idealized therapist, which can serve as a corrective emotional experience (Alexander and French 1946). However, certain types of patients, such as help-rejecting complainers (see Chapter 5, "General Framework of Supportive Psychotherapy"), will maintain a transference position that is impermeable to therapist intervention and disclosure. Moreover, their pathogenic beliefs regarding self and others are confirmed by the therapist's repeated attempts to engage and problem solve (Sampson and Weiss 1986).

# 7

# Crisis Intervention

## History and Theory

Crisis intervention began during World War II out of a necessity to treat soldiers exposed to battlefield conditions. In World War I, soldiers with combat fatigue or shell shock (now called traumatic stress disorder) were quickly evacuated from the front lines, without treatment, despite observations that early intervention might reduce psychiatric morbidity (Salmon 1919). These soldiers often regressed or even became chronically impaired. In World War II, soldiers were treated at or near the front lines with crisis intervention techniques and were quickly returned to their combat units (Glass 1954).

At about the same time, Lindemann (1944) began working with survivors and relatives of survivors of the Coconut Grove nightclub fire in Boston, individuals in acute grief who were unable to cope with their bereavement. In his seminal article, Lindemann (1944) described normal and morbid grief and contrasted the two. The survivors and their families were helped to do the necessary "grief work," which involved going through the mourning process and experiencing the loss. One of Lindemann's colleagues, Gerald Caplan (1961), began to work in the field of preventive psychiatry and helped develop the theoretical basis for the community mental health movement. Lindemann and Caplan were among the most important early theoreticians of the crisis intervention approach.

Parad and Parad (1990) defined *crisis* as an "upset in a steady state, a turning point leading to better or worse, a disruption or breakdown in a person's or family's normal or usual pattern of functioning" (pp. 3–4). A crisis occurs when an individual encounters a situation that leads to a breakdown in his or her usual pattern of functioning, creating disequilibrium. Generally, a crisis is precipitated by a hazardous event or a stressor, such as a catastrophe or disaster (e.g., an earthquake, a fire, war, or terrorism), a relationship rupture or loss, rape, or abuse. A crisis may also result from a series of difficult events or mishaps rather than from one major occurrence, and a crisis can be a response to external and internal stress. During crisis, individuals perceive their lives, needs, security, relationships, and sense of well-being to be at risk. Crises tend to be time limited, generally lasting no more than a few months; the duration depends on the stressor and on the individual's perception of and response to the stressor.

Crisis states can lead to personal growth rather than physical and psychological deterioration (Caplan 1961). Growth is possible because the crisis assaults the individual's psychic structure and defenses, throwing them into a state of flux, which can make the individual more open to treatment. Davanloo (1980) incorporated production of a crisis into his short-term dynamic psychotherapy approach, as a means of disrupting ingrained defenses in order for patients to gain access to their inner lives and thereby change maladaptive ways of feeling, thinking, and behaving.

Crisis intervention is a therapeutic process aimed at restoring homeostatic balance and diminishing vulnerability to the stressor. Homeostasis is accomplished by the therapist's helping to mobilize the individual's abilities and social network and to promote adaptive coping mechanisms to reestablish equilibrium. Crisis intervention is a short-term approach that focuses on solving the immediate problem and includes the entire therapeutic repertoire for helping patients deal with the challenges and threats of overwhelming stress.

An individual's reaction to stress is the result of a number of factors, including age, health, personality issues, prior experience with stressful events, support and belief systems, and underlying biological or genetic vulnerability. Traumatic events are common and varied and can be personal, such as the death of a loved one, rape, the experience of being robbed, or involvement in a traffic accident. Other types of trauma, such as natural disasters or terrorist attacks, may involve large numbers of individuals, including persons not on the scene. In addition, the intensity and type of traumatic event are also important, as is an individual's coping ability. At times, a series of traumatic events may produce a crisis that a single event would not have provoked. An example might be a series of losses resulting in a crisis that did not occur after the first few losses.

Losses include death, separation, illness, financial loss, and loss of employment, function, or status.

The distinction between crisis intervention and psychotherapy is often blurred, because the approaches may overlap with regard to technique and length of treatment. Crisis intervention is generally expected to involve one to three contacts, and the duration of brief psychotherapy can extend from a few visits to 20 or more sessions. In this chapter, the term *crisis intervention* is also used for crisis-related treatment lasting longer than just a few sessions. This more inclusive form of crisis therapy is based on a number of different treatments, including dynamic supportive, cognitive-behavioral, humanistic, family, and systems approaches, as well as the use of medication when indicated. Systems approaches can be broad and can encompass actions such as working with and referral to social service agencies, clergy, mobile crisis units, suicide hotlines, and law enforcement agencies. In recent years, the focus of crisis intervention has been on emergency management and prevention through the use of various forms of debriefing.

## Evaluation

According to Caplan (1961), ego assessment (see Chapter 4, "Assessment, Case Formulation, Goal Setting, and Outcome Research") is the key in the evaluation of an individual in a crisis situation. The evaluation consists of 1) examining the individual's capacity to deal with stress, maintain ego structure and equilibrium, and deal with reality and 2) assessing problem-solving and coping abilities.

The evaluation of an individual in a crisis situation should be thorough and systematic but should also be essentially completed within the first session. A timely evaluation is critical, to enable the therapist to develop a case formulation and treatment plan and initiate treatment immediately. Indeed, even the evaluation session should be therapeutic, because the patient is in crisis and is seeking relief from suffering. The evaluation should follow the process outlined in Chapter 4, but should focus on the traumatic situation, precipitating event, and possible danger to self and others. The individual's experience of the trauma, including perceptions and feelings, is important, as is whether the person was a victim or a witness of the traumatic event. Also, the therapist should assess 1) the individual's current affect, anxiety level, and sense of hopefulness and 2) the way in which he or she attempts to deal with the trauma.

The following case example illustrates the evaluation process in a broad-based, supportive psychotherapy/crisis intervention approach.

## Case Vignette

William is a 44-year-old police officer with anxiety, depressive feelings, an inability to work, and difficulty enjoying anything about his life. He is tall, muscular, and physically imposing. In his first session, he reveals that he recently had a traumatic experience.

### Session 1

Therapist: What is troubling you?

William: I've been having all kinds of problems. I can't work... can't sleep....I don't enjoy anything in my life anymore. (**Responds with multiple complaints**)

Therapist: So you are having trouble working and sleeping and are not finding enjoyment in your life. How long have you been having these difficulties? (**Summarizes and attempts to find out when William's difficulties began**)

William: About 6 months, but it's gotten worse during the last couple of months.

Therapist: I see, your problems began 6 months ago. What was happening in your life at that time? (**Begins to focus on the beginning of the episode of illness**)

William: Nine-eleven happened. I was sent down there right at the beginning with three other cops. It was terrible. I still can't believe what happened. (**Begins to talk about the traumatic events that occurred on September 11, 2001**)

Therapist: It's important that we go into this in some detail. Can you tell me what occurred when you arrived at the World Trade Center? (**Attempts to get details of the traumatic event and its effect on William**)

William: I was told to wait outside, and the others went in. They never came out....I should have been there with them. [begins to cry] (**Is filled with emotion and perhaps feelings of guilt**)

Therapist: This is very difficult for you. (**Responds in an empathic manner**)

William: Yeah. I was told to stay outside and monitor traffic, not allow any civilians in. So I stayed out there.

Therapist: You were outside, and they went in, and then what happened?

William: Well, I was standing there....I looked up....I saw people jumping. I was stunned.

Therapist: My God! That must have been...frightening. (**Responds with emotion and in an empathic manner**)

William: Yeah....I saw a man and a woman jumping...holding hands...[begins to sob] (**Responds with further information**)

Therapist: You went through a terrible ordeal. What a horror! (**Responds empathically**)

William: That's only the first part of it. Then all of a sudden, the building began to come down, and I ran. I was buried, and I couldn't see.

Then I saw my wife and son holding hands and waving to me....I thought I was dead.

Therapist: You were buried, and you saw your wife and son. You thought you were dead. How did you get through that experience? (***Responds with a clarification, tracking, and admiration and continues exploring***)

William: I was paralyzed at first...couldn't reason. I felt like a mummy.... I didn't move right away.

Therapist: Then what?

William: Then I reached for my eyes, and I pulled out stuff from around my eyes and ears, and I stood up and realized I was alive. I don't know how I got out....I saw a woman next to me buried, trying to get up, so I pulled stuff off her and picked her up and carried her to a rescue area. Then I went back and got a man and carried him out. (***Despite his horrendous ordeal, William behaved in a heroic manner.***)

Therapist: You helped save two people! After what you went through, you rescued two people! (***Praises and expresses admiration for William for his heroic behavior***)

William: Yes, but I...the cops I came with...they never got out. I should have been there with them. I keep thinking about it. (***Despite his heroic behavior and the therapist's praise and admiration, William indicates that he feels guilty about not going in with the other policemen.***)

Therapist: You were a hero, yet you still believe that you should have been with them. Losing three fellow officers must have been devastating. (***Begins to address the issue of William surviving while his fellow officers all died***)

This vignette illustrates part of the process of evaluating a patient who is in a crisis situation and has a traumatic stress disorder. In the remainder of the evaluation, the therapist explores William's guilt about staying behind while others went in, his level of anxiety, and the extent of his depression. William's current family situation is examined, as well as his history. The following information emerges:

The patient has been extremely anxious and tearful following his traumatic experience. He has been pacing back and forth in his home and thinking constantly about what happened to him on September 11, 2001. He has startle reactions to loud noises and has flashbacks about the building collapsing, people jumping, and seeing his wife and son. William has nightmares and so avoids sleep. He can no longer concentrate, has little energy, feels helpless, and no longer enjoys anything in his life. The patient has been unable to return to work and tries to avoid anything that might remind him of September 11. His previous performance at work was quite good, and he was decorated on several occasions for heroism.

William grew up in a middle class family and had a good relationship with his mother. When the patient was 15 years old, his father died. William's relationship with his father had been difficult and filled with conflict, which resulted in mixed feelings toward his father. These feelings did not resolve when the patient's father was dying, and they may have played a role in William's emphasis on bodybuilding and on presenting a strong, manly image.

The therapist concludes that William has posttraumatic stress disorder. Before the trauma, the patient was functioning at a high level and had good coping skills, despite unresolved problems with his father. At present, his coping skills are no longer adequate, but he has a supportive spouse and appears to be motivated for psychotherapy. The treatment goals, formulated with the patient, include amelioration of his symptoms and return to work. The treatment plan includes development of a supportive, positive therapeutic relationship at the onset of treatment, followed by work on symptom reduction with the use of exposure therapy, along with cognitive restructuring. Medication for his anxiety and depression, such as a selective serotonin reuptake inhibitor, may also be indicated. As treatment progresses, a major focus will be to help the patient return to work as soon as possible.

## Treatment

The therapeutic approaches used in crisis intervention are primarily those of brief supportive psychotherapy, consisting of maintenance of focus and a high therapist-activity level; use of clearly established goals, a time limit, and a number of supportive and cognitive-behavioral interventions; and, most importantly, establishment of a solid therapeutic alliance. There are a number of systematic approaches to crisis intervention (James and Gilliland 2001; Puryear 1979; Roberts 2000).

Systematic approaches to crisis intervention all stress assessment, patient safety, establishment of rapport and hopefulness, supportive interventions, and positive actions and plans. The importance of assessment was discussed in the previous section, "Evaluation." Patient safety is part of the assessment process and should be monitored throughout therapy if the individual's safety is in question (see discussion in "Suicide" later in this chapter). Establishing rapport and promoting hopefulness are important in all forms of psychotherapy and are major factors in fostering the therapeutic alliance. The therapeutic alliance has been shown to be the best predictor of success in psychotherapy (Gaston 1990; Horvath and Symonds 1991). The major elements of the alliance (Gaston 1990) are the patient's affective bond with the therapist, the patient's ability to work purposefully and collaboratively with the therapist, the therapist's empathic understanding and involvement, and the agreement of patient and therapist on the goals and tasks of therapy. The use of supportive or empathic interventions helps promote the alliance, making it possible to use exposure techniques to help resolve the patient's reaction to the trauma. Positive actions and plans provide the patient with structure and improve self-esteem and hope for the future. The following case example illustrates the treatment process in a broad-based supportive psychotherapy crisis intervention approach.

## Case Vignette (continued)

William (the police officer with posttraumatic stress disorder resulting from the events of September 11, 2001) has completed his first session of supportive psychotherapy/crisis intervention (see "Case Vignette" in previous section). In addition, treatment with a selective serotonin reuptake inhibitor has been started, with the dose gradually being increased to a therapeutic level during the course of treatment. The next two sessions are primarily directed at forming a secure and positive therapeutic alliance through the use of supportive interventions. Part of the patient's second session follows.

### Session 2

William: My wife told me that I don't bother with her anymore, that I just ignore her...but I don't feel like doing anything....I don't feel like talking. (**Begins with a complaint from his wife rather than continuing with the traumatic event; response may be defensive**)

Therapist: Last week at our first meeting, we explored what happened to you on that terrible day, something about your past life, and a bit about your relationship with your wife and son. Let's look at your current relationship with your wife. (**Chooses to address William's current issue with his wife, the intention being to build a therapeutic relationship before going back to the traumatic event, which William may not be ready for at the current time**)

William: Well...Cathy comes over to me and tries to talk to me...get me started talking, but I don't feel like talking; it's too much. (**Indicates that he is overwhelmed, which may have implications for his feelings about talking to the therapist**)

Therapist: So it's hard for you to talk. Perhaps there are some things that would be easier for you to talk about. (**Responds in an empathic manner and asks William to focus on areas that are less painful, anxiety provoking, and conflictual**)

William: It's hard to talk about 9/11...but I like to talk about my son, things to do with our house...and the garden.

Therapist: So you could talk with Cathy about these things—the house and your son. Can you give me an example of what you might feel comfortable talking to Cathy about?

The therapist has recognized that the patient is having difficulty talking at home and is possibly having difficulty talking with the therapist. However, because the patient is talking spontaneously, the therapist has decided not to address the therapeutic relationship and instead has begun to focus on concrete areas that the patient can discuss with his wife. Focusing on concrete areas helps to reduce anxiety, which is important in both supportive psychotherapy and crisis intervention:

William: Cathy wants to send Billy to summer camp. I don't know—he's not much of an athlete, but he likes to play the saxophone. Maybe it's better if he stays home. (***Indicates his wish to have Billy at home with him***)
Therapist: Could it be that you disagree with Cathy because you would like to have Billy at home? (***Tentatively asks William if he disagrees with Cathy about sending Billy to camp***)
William: I like to have him around. (***Ignores his conflict with Cathy and focuses on Billy***)
Therapist: So would I be correct in saying that you want Billy to be with you but you find it hard to talk to Cathy directly about what you think? (***Brings William back to his conflict with Cathy; using a supportive approach, asks if he agrees***)
William: That makes sense. I just can't be clear about what I want, because I really don't know. (***Agrees but indicates that he becomes passive and indecisive with Cathy***)
Therapist: It sounds like you would like to have Billy home this summer, but it's hard for you to be direct with Cathy, so you hang back and get distracted and annoyed with her. Do you agree? (***Interprets William's wish to have Billy home and William's defensive posture of passivity and distraction accompanied by annoyance with Cathy; again employs the supportive technique of asking for feedback so that William is not overwhelmed***)

The therapist has asked for a specific example of William's difficulty in communicating with his wife. Obtaining specific concrete examples from patients is always preferable to leaving things on a general level. When patients generalize, it is difficult to understand what they have in mind. In addition, it is not helpful to patients to remain in a confused or unclear state.

Having understood that William wishes to have his son at home, the therapist has been able to clarify this wish with William. The therapist has used a number of supportive approaches. Instead of addressing allusions to the transference, the therapist has continued to concentrate on the patient's current life and his difficulty with Cathy. In supportive psychotherapy, the transference generally is not addressed unless it is negative. Instead, the therapist concentrates on current issues in the patient's life and on the real relationship with the therapist. Clarification is useful as a supportive technique because it does not place demands or therapist expectations on the patient. In addition, the therapist has been able to link William's avoidance and annoyance with his wife to his wish to keep Billy home for the summer and not have him go off to camp as his wife wishes.

The pursuit of affect is generally avoided in supportive psychotherapy and has been avoided in this session. However, William's emotional experiences resulting from the World Trade Center tragedy will need to be addressed when exposure techniques are used later in therapy.

## Session 4

The therapist has determined that a good therapeutic relationship was established during the first three sessions. Therefore, exposure therapy within a supportive framework can now be attempted to enable the patient to work through his traumatic experience:

Therapist: I thought that we might go back and explore what happened to you on 9/11. If we can look at your experience together, it should help you to better deal with it and move on with your life. How do you feel about doing that now? (*Asks for William's agreement to explore his traumatic experience. Asking for agreement constitutes the supportive technique of agenda setting.*)

William: If it can help....I think I'm more ready.

Therapist: It's good that you feel ready and able to proceed. Let's go back to that day when you went to the World Trade Center, OK? (*Praises William*)

William: OK.

Therapist: You and your fellow officers were sent to the World Trade Center about when? (*Begins a detailed exploration of William's traumatic experience*)

William: In the morning, after the second plane hit...we drove up.

Therapist: And as you drove up, what were you experiencing?

William: The fires were raging....We knew by then it was an attack. The sergeant said I should stay outside and keep people out.

Therapist: What was it like for you, remaining outside while the others went in? (*Is aware of William's not wanting to remain behind and his guilt feelings about being the only survivor from his group*)

William: I wanted to go with them.

Therapist: So you felt...? (*For the first time, the therapist asks about William's feelings. Exposure therapy relies on the patient's experiencing and exploring feelings, in a somewhat controlled fashion, during the session.*)

> William: I felt useless…annoyed. I didn't want to stay behind.
> Therapist: That's understandable, but you were ordered to stay behind.

The therapist has emphasized that William was ordered to stay behind, because during the evaluation session, William indicated that he felt guilty and conflicted about waiting outside. The therapist is preparing the groundwork for addressing William's cognitive distortion of this issue and his possible survivor guilt.

The session continues with a recounting of the traumatic events that followed:

> William: I was standing there…in the street. Then all of a sudden, I saw people jumping from the building. Some of them were on fire.
> Therapist: That's horrible! What were you feeling? (***Asks William for his feelings in an empathic manner***)
> William: It was hard to look….[*begins to sob*] I couldn't believe it. Then I saw a man and a woman jumping…holding hands…[*becomes visibly shaken and anxious*]
> Therapist: Who wouldn't be devastated, shaken, and tearful? (***Clarifies in an empathic manner using the supportive technique of normalizing***)

The therapist has been obtaining a detailed account of William's traumatic experience and has also been monitoring the patient's level of anxiety so that the anxiety will remain within manageable limits. If a patient's anxiety level gets too high, the therapist can slow down the account and initiate anxiety-lowering interventions, such as having the patient engage in progressive muscular relaxation and deep breathing. In addition to these techniques, which are generally used in exposure therapy, supportive interventions such as reassurance can be used.

The session continues with a detailed exploration of the patient's experiences of that day, including the collapse of the buildings, near burial in the debris, hallucination of his wife and son, and his belief that he was dead. The therapist elicits these experiences in great detail and in an empathic manner, with careful monitoring of the patient's anxiety level. During the exploration of William's vision of his wife and son, the vision in which he saw them holding hands and waving goodbye to him, William becomes visibly shaken and anxious because at that time he believed he was dead. The therapist stops the exploration and begins anxiety-lowering approaches, including progressive muscular relaxation and deep breathing.

## Session 5

The session begins with a discussion of the patient's anxiety level during the interval between sessions. This information is important because the aim in supportive therapy is to keep the anxiety level as low as possible. William indicates that he has not been experiencing a significant amount of anxiety:

> Therapist: Do you feel ready now to continue exploring what happened to you on 9/11? (**Checks to see if William is ready to continue exposure therapy; again uses the supportive technique of agenda setting**)
> William: Yeah…I can keep going.
> Therapist: You have strength and resilience. Let's pick up where we left off: after you saw your wife and son. Is that OK? (**Offers praise— a supportive intervention—and then resumes exploration of William's traumatic experience**)
> William: Yeah, I began to realize that maybe I wasn't dead, and I started to push away all the stuff covering me…around my eyes, in my ears, all over me. (**Continues without much difficulty**)
> Therapist: So you began to realize you were not dead and felt how?
> Patient: I felt some relief.…I thought, Thank God, I think I'm all right. Then I got up and saw a woman on her knees. She was bleeding from her scalp. I helped her up and carried her to a rescue area.
> Therapist: So despite your being battered and thinking you were dead a few minutes earlier, you were able to pull a woman out of the rubble and rescue her! (**Offers praise and expresses admiration— both useful supportive interventions, provided the praise and admiration are clearly reality based and deserved**)

The therapist goes on to explore the details of the patient's next few hours after he picked himself up from the rubble. These details include rescuing a man, going to the hospital to have lacerations sutured, and finding out that the three policemen who went into the building died. All these experiences are fully explored during the next few sessions, until William can talk about his experience without too much anxiety or overwhelming sadness.

William's treatment involves the use of exposure therapy in the context of a supportive relationship. The therapist is able to take the patient through his traumatic experience in a slow and detailed manner over the course of several meetings. The therapist monitors William's anxiety level so that he is not overwhelmed. If the patient begins to become overly aroused, the therapist stops the exposure work and uses a number of supportive techniques, such as praise, reassurance, and relaxation therapy. At the same time, a great deal of work is required to restructure William's excessive feeling of guilt about being the only survivor of his group of four policemen. The therapist challenges William's self-blaming cognitions, to help him reframe his idea that he should have been inside the World Trade Center with his fellow officers. The therapist helps William understand the concept of survivor guilt when he states, "Many people who survive tragedies as you did feel guilty."

After 10 sessions, William gradually improves and is able to return to work and to feel comfortable with his wife and son. He still has episodes of anxiety and sadness, which he is able to manage, and he continues taking medication. He has two follow-up sessions, 1 month later and then 3 months later, to prevent relapse.

# Suicide

The prediction of suicide is problematic because there is no reliable way of determining suicidal risk in a given individual (Fawcett 1993; Pokorny 1983). Two major problems occur when attempts are made to predict suicide: identification of too many false-positive cases, and oversight of many instances of completed suicide. However, it is known that more than 90% of completed suicides occur in individuals with a recent major psychiatric illness. The most common diagnoses are major depression, chronic alcoholism and drug abuse, schizophrenia, borderline personality disorder, bipolar disorder, and eating disorders. A careful and thorough assessment of the suicidal patient is critical to determine the diagnosis and the proper treatment approach. Crisis intervention approaches, generally accompanied by the use of medication, often play an important role in the treatment of suicidal individuals.

## Assessment of Risk

Suicidal thoughts and behaviors are so common that it is essential to ask all patients about suicidal ideas and attempts. A history of suicide attempts increases a person's risk for suicide. Individuals who have well-defined plans to kill themselves are at greater risk than individuals with vague or poorly formulated plans. When a suicidal person has the means to end his or her life (e.g., owns a firearm), the patient is at significant risk. The presence of strong family support or a significant other can have a mitigating effect on suicidal risk. Hopelessness, pessimism, aggression, impulsiveness, and psychic anxiety are poor prognostic signs. Another factor to be considered is the loss of a significant other through separation, divorce, or death.

Paradoxically, it has been found that more than half of patients who died by suicide had consulted clinicians within one year before death and had denied suicidal thoughts or indicated that they rarely occurred (Clark and Fawcett 1992). Often, these same patients communicated directly or indirectly to a close friend or relative that they were thinking of ending their lives. This information suggests that physicians should routinely question close relatives and friends of patients who may be at risk for suicide.

Fawcett and colleagues (1990, 1993) divided suicidal risk into acute and chronic categories. Individuals who are at acute risk often have severe anxiety, thoughts about negative events occurring, insomnia, anhedonia, agitation, and alcohol abuse (Busch et al. 2003). Persons at more chronic risk have more-typical risk factors, such as suicidal ideation and plans, and a history of suicide attempts.

The risk of suicide is often greatest during the week after hospital admission and the month after discharge and during the early period of recovery from a psychiatric disorder (Hawton 1987).

## Treatment

Once it has been determined that an individual is acutely suicidal, hospitalization may be indicated. If hospitalization is not feasible or not absolutely necessary, it is important to enlist the aid of significant others, who can spend time with the patient and not leave the patient alone. The therapist needs to make himself or herself available for contact either by the patient or by the patient's family or friends. Information regarding 24-hour hotlines and the nearest emergency room should be given to the suicidal patient and family or friends. Medication is often necessary to relieve anxiety, agitation, or depression. The frequency of treatment sessions will vary, depending on the patient's needs. Some patients may need to be seen daily, for ongoing support and structure. Accordingly, it is important that the same clinician see the patient throughout the period of crisis intervention. Important issues to focus on are patient hopelessness and pessimism. Supportive approaches involving praise, reassurance, and cognitive restructuring are often useful to help enhance self-esteem by counteracting negative or distorted cognitions about the self. As always, establishment and maintenance of a positive therapeutic alliance are essential.

## Crisis Intervention Versus Psychotherapy

As stated in "History and Theory" at the beginning of this chapter, crisis intervention theory is based on a number of psychological approaches, including dynamic supportive psychotherapy, cognitive-behavioral therapy, humanistic treatments, family therapy, and systems approaches.

Crisis intervention is time limited and is not focused on psychological insight, personality issues, or psychiatric disorders. An individual receiving crisis intervention is generally in transition or has lost his or her equilibrium because of a traumatic experience that has disrupted his or her life. The objective is to help the individual deal with the stressful period, achieve stability, and return to his or her precrisis level of functioning or, if the patient needs further treatment, move on to the next level of care.

Crisis intervention differs from psychotherapy in a number of ways (outlined in Table 7–1). Crisis treatment is given as soon as possible and in close proximity to the stressor or traumatic event. It is time limited, and the therapist is active, supportive, and directive. As in supportive psychotherapy, the focus is on the here and now rather than on the past or on transference issues.

## Critical Incident Stress Management

Critical incident stress management (CISM) was originally developed for use with emergency workers. More recently, however, its scope has been expanded to include anyone exposed to severe trauma (Everly and Mitchell 1999; Mitchell and Everly 2003). CISM is a comprehensive and integrated crisis intervention approach for individuals and groups. The components of CISM are summarized in Table 7–2 and include the following: precrisis preparation involving stress management education and training, for individuals and groups of professional and emergency workers; briefings on disasters and terrorist or other large-scale incidents, for rescue workers and civilians; defusing (i.e., immediate small-group discussion), to ensure assessment and triage and to mitigate symptoms; critical incident stress debriefing (CISD) (Mitchell and Everly 1996), to reduce impairments from traumatic stress, facilitate closure, and mitigate symptoms, for individuals and groups; individual or family crisis intervention; and follow-up and referral for further assessment and treatment.

A component of CISM, a typical CISD approach after a traumatic event involves a group of victims who undergo the stages, just described above, in a single 1- to 3-hour session. The efficacy of a single-session debriefing in preventing posttraumatic stress disorder or other disorders has recently come into question. In a meta-analysis of single-session debriefing within 1 month after trauma, van Emmerik and colleagues (2002) found that CISD interventions do not improve natural recovery from psychological trauma. It may be that single-session approaches of this sort help reduce immediate distress and provide for referral for further treatment. Positive outcomes have been achieved with cognitive-behav-

**Table 7–1.** Crisis intervention versus psychotherapy

| | Crisis intervention | Psychotherapy |
|---|---|---|
| Context | Prevention | Reparation |
| Timing | Immediate; close temporal relationship to stressor or acute decompensation | Delayed; distant from stressor or acute decompensation |
| Location | Close proximity to stressor or acute decompensation; anywhere needed | Safe, secure environment |
| Duration | Typically one to three contacts | As long as needed or desired |
| Provider's role | Active, directive | Guiding, collaborative, consultative |
| Strategic foci | Conscious processes, environmental stressors or factors | Conscious and unconscious sources of pathogenesis |
| Temporal focus | Here and now | Present and past |
| Patient expectations | Symptom reduction, reduction of impairment, directive support | Symptom reduction, reduction of impairment, personal growth, guidance, collaboration |
| Goals | Stabilization, reduction of impairment, a return to function or a shift to next level of care | Symptom reduction, reduction of impairment, correction of pathogenesis, personal growth, personal reconstruction |

*Source.* Aguilera et al. 1970; Artiss 1963; Everly and Mitchell 1998; Koss and Shiang 1994; Salmon 1919; Sandoval 1985; Skaikeu 1990; Spiegel and Classen 1995; Wilkinson and Vera 1985.
Reprinted from Everly GS Jr, Mitchell JT: *Critical Incident Stress Management (CISM): A New Era and Standard of Care in Crisis Intervention.* Ellicott City, MD, Chevron Publishing, 1999. Used with permission.

**Table 7–2.** Core components of critical incident stress management

| Intervention | Timing | Activation | Goals | Recipients |
|---|---|---|---|---|
| Precrisis preparation | Precrisis | Driven by crisis anticipation | Setting of expectations, improved coping, stress management | Individuals, groups, organizations |
| Demobilization and staff consultation (rescuers) | Shift disengagement | Event driven | Presentation of information, consultation, psychological decompression, stress management | Organizations, large groups |
| Crisis management briefing (civilians, schools, businesses) | Anytime postcrisis | Event driven | Presentation of information, consultation, psychological decompression, stress management | Organizations, large groups |
| Defusing | Postcrisis (within 12 hours) | Usually symptom driven | Symptom mitigation, possible closure, triage | Small groups |
| Critical incident stress debriefing | Postcrisis (1–10 days; mass disasters: 3–4 weeks) | Usually symptom driven; sometimes event driven | Facilitation of psychological closure, symptom mitigation, triage | Individuals, small groups |
| Individual crisis intervention | Anytime, anywhere | Symptom driven | Symptom mitigation, possible return to function, referral if needed | Individuals |
| Family crisis intervention | Anytime | Symptom or event driven | Fostering of support and communication | Families |

**Table 7–2.** Core components of critical incident stress management (*continued*)

| Intervention | Timing | Activation | Goals | Recipients |
|---|---|---|---|---|
| Community and organizational consultation | Anytime | Symptom or event driven | Symptom mitigation, possible closure, referral if needed | Organizations |
| Pastoral crisis intervention | Anytime | Usually symptom driven | "Crisis of faith" mitigation, use of spiritual tools to assist in recovery | Individuals, families, groups |
| Follow-up and referral | Anytime | Usually symptom driven | Mental status assessment, a shift to higher level of care if needed | Individuals, families |

*Source.* Adapted from Everly GS Jr, Mitchell JT: *Critical Incident Stress Management (CISM): A New Era and Standard of Care in Crisis Intervention.* Ellicott City, MD, Chevron Publishing, 1999. Used with permission.

ioral treatments that were administered within the first month of the traumatic incident and that involved education, exposure, and cognitive restructuring (Bryant et al. 1999; Foa 1997; Foa et al. 1991).

## Summary

In this chapter, we provided a brief history and the theoretical background of crisis intervention. Individuals exposed to severe trauma can react in a number of ways, and some of these reactions necessitate crisis intervention. A thorough evaluation of a patient presenting in crisis is always necessary. Treatment approaches used vary depending on the needs of the patient but generally include supportive interventions, exposure therapy, and cognitive restructuring. Therapists must pay particular attention to establishing and maintaining a positive therapeutic alliance. The terrorist attacks of September 11, 2001, in New York and Washington, DC, have made both the general public and mental health professionals more aware of these issues and the need for crisis intervention services.

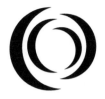

# 8

# Applicability to Special Populations

## Severe Mental Illness

As originally conceived, supportive psychotherapy was indicated for patients with severe mental illness, as well as for other patients for whom expressive treatment was not indicated. That supportive psychotherapy approach was the treatment at the extreme supportive end of the supportive-expressive psychotherapy continuum described in Chapter 1, "Basic Principles of Supportive Psychotherapy." This form of supportive treatment was focused mainly on optimizing deficient ego functions, reducing anxiety, and preventing downward social drift due to loss of adaptive skills and increasing isolation. In addition to offering the patient the contact of an understanding, supportive relationship, this approach consisted mainly of the following techniques: advice, reassurance, exhortation, praise, encouragement, "lending ego," and environmental manipulation. Shoring up of defenses was the default mode, confrontation was rare, and interpretation did not occur.

Today, we know that even for patients who are quite impaired because of severe mental illness, there should be a balance between supportive and expressive elements in supportive treatment. Depending on several factors—including the degree of stabilization after acute exacerbation of illness, the strength of the therapeutic alliance (see Chapter 6, "The Therapeutic Relationship"), and the patient's treatment goals—confrontation and, at times, interpretation can be useful techniques in supportive psychotherapy. Cognitive learning strategies such as teaching, using slogans, modeling, and giving anticipatory guidance are commonly used. The treatment components of psychoeducation and skills training, which have been framed as independent interventions, are consistent with the model of supportive treatment and are particularly useful in supportive psychotherapy for chronic mental illness.

## Schizophrenia

Schizophrenia is the prototypical severe mental illness. When treating a patient who has schizophrenia, the therapist provides education about the illness, promotes medication compliance, facilitates reality testing, encourages problem solving by the patient, and reinforces adaptive behavior with praise (Lamberti and Herz 1995). Gunderson and colleagues (1984) demonstrated that patients with schizophrenia have better treatment retention and better outcome when given weekly supportive treatment as compared to more intensive expressive treatment.

Praise is a form of reinforcement that can support the patient's self-esteem and motivation for adaptive change. As described in detail in Chapter 3, "Interventions (What to Say)," praise is an important esteem-building technique. However, praise builds self-esteem only when the praised behavior is considered praiseworthy by the patient. Thus, the therapist must understand what the patient will find worthy of praise. It is also important for the therapist to attempt to understand what the patient finds rewarding besides praise, so that these incentives can be enlisted in order to provide positive feedback. Determining what the patient finds rewarding is especially important at the left side of the psychopathology continuum (e.g., in schizophrenia), where positive reinforcement is an important factor in maintaining the therapeutic alliance and motivating engagement in treatment. Positive reinforcement is helpful for patients with schizophrenia because they commonly have neurocognitive impairments; negative symptoms, such as apathy, anhedonia, and poor motivation; and poor insight. A reinforcer can be a favorite food, activity, person, or social event that increases the strength or frequency of the patient's contingent behavior. Properly assessed and delivered reinforcers increase patients' skill acquisition, achievement of goals, and self-esteem (Lecomte et al. 2000). External rewards that patients value may be helpful for engaging and maintaining these patients in treatment. These rewards can include subway tokens, certificates of accomplishment, a celebratory event, and gift certificates. Administration of accurate praise, as described throughout this book, is an effective and inexpensive reward.

## Psychoeducation

Typically, supportive psychotherapy for patients with severe mental illness includes psychoeducation about the illness, its trajectory, and its treatment. The literature suggests that educating patients about their schizophrenia or substance dependence reinforces psychosocial rehabilitation (Goldman and Quinn 1988). Most patients find learning new information to be generally supportive. When provided in an empathic way, psychoeducation offers the patient a new cognitive structure on which to base more-realistic decision making. Psychoeducation also gives the patient an explanation of or rationale for symptoms and suffering; giving such explanations or rationales may also bolster the patient's self-esteem.

In addition, concrete information about the illness arms the patient with practical knowledge that can help improve his or her ability to cope with chronic illness—an adaptive skill. For example, early in an exacerbation of the manic phase of bipolar disorder, the patient frequently loses the capacity to understand that his or her judgment is impaired by mania. During a remission, the psychiatrist can teach the patient that sleeping even an hour less than usual for two nights in a row may be an early sign of relapse to mania. This information gives the patient an opportunity to demonstrate some adaptive mastery over the illness and act before an exacerbation can impair judgment acutely and destroy the chance to "step on the brakes." When the symptom of impaired sleep occurs, and the patient contacts the psychiatrist for a dose escalation of antimania medications, the patient will likely experience increased self-efficacy and an increase in self-esteem. These positive effects will occur as a result of the patient's sense of increased competence in anticipating potentially damaging future events and will strengthen the therapeutic alliance.

## Supporting Adaptive Skills

To help patients who have impairments in interpersonal functioning and severe mental disorders such as schizophrenia, behavioral skills training and other cognitive-behavioral techniques can be integrated into supportive psychotherapy. The model of change in supportive therapy is change through learning and introjection or identification with an accepting, well-related therapist (Pinsker et al. 1991). Training in social and independent-living skills for severely mentally ill patients is an approach grounded in learning principles, wherein the therapist breaks down complex social repertoires and models correct behavior for the patient, who repeatedly practices the skills after learning them. After the steps are assembled, the patient practices the complex interaction—first with the therapist, then in the real world. The therapist uses supportive techniques such as behavioral-goal setting, encouragement, modeling, shaping, and praise (positive reinforcement) to teach the interpersonal skills (Glynn et al. 2002). This activity directly supports adaptive skills and builds patients' self-esteem. Studies have demonstrated the utility of these interventions in improving social competence (Heinssen et al. 2000; Lauriello et al. 1999). Patients with schizophrenia have deficits in social skills, which may be a result of impaired information processing. Skills training uses the problem-solving, repetitive, and practical approach of supportive psychotherapy and is effective in improving basic conversational skills, recreational skills, medication management, and management of symptoms (Liberman et al. 1998; Smith et al. 1999). A related cognitive-behavioral approach, relapse prevention, is discussed in "Adaptive Skills and Relapse Prevention" later in this chapter.

At times, the clinician must balance his or her focus on anxiety reduction as a major supportive strategy against the patient's determination to work through a particular problem, which could increase the patient's adaptive skills. For example, a patient might become anxious on hearing details about schizophrenia. However, providing guidance about hearing the information, and reframing the content in an attempt to shore up the patient's coping skills, might reduce the patient's anxiety. Having more extensive coping strategies that use higher-level defenses (e.g., rationalization) can mean that the patient has a more flexible and adaptive approach to his or her illness. At other times, when the patient signals that there is too much anxiety to deal with a subject directly, it can be useful for the therapist to attempt to "back into" discussion of the difficult topic:

Therapist: So, Mr. Green, I would like to talk to you about what you understand about your illness. Is that OK with you? (*"Shows the map" before exploring the territory*)
Patient: I guess.
Therapist: If what I'm saying doesn't make sense to you, please tell me and I'll try to clarify it. If it just makes you more nervous, let me know, and we'll talk about something else. OK? (*Offers anticipatory guidance about material to be explored, gives the patient permission to stop the exploration, sets a collaborative tone, and indicates that the therapist is sensitive to the patient's feelings.*)
Patient: All right.
Therapist: Has anyone discussed with you what your diagnosis is? That means the medical name of the illness that's bringing you into psychiatric treatment.
Patient: Uh, depression. I have depression.
Therapist: That's what they told you?
Patient: I don't know....Um, I have depression. (*The patient has been*

*told previously that his diagnosis is schizophrenia. He is either being evasive or using denial.*)

Therapist: Could you describe for me what the word *depression* means to you?

Patient: Yeah, I couldn't sleep, and I don't do much. Don't feel like it. I used to do things.

Therapist: Any other problems, like in your thoughts or feelings?

Patient: I have depression. (*Concrete, perseverative, nonelaborative answer*)

Therapist: Are you sad a lot? People who are depressed are often sad.

Patient: No, not sad. I just don't feel much of anything. Tired. I don't know. (*Disclaims a low mood associated with depression*)

Therapist: OK. Now, other than being tired, are there things you've been experiencing lately that have caused you problems?

Patient: Huh? Like what? [*suspicious look*]

Therapist: Well, you told the other doctor back in your intake evaluation that you had been thinking that somebody or maybe some group was trying to harm you, that you saw evidence of that. Is that accurate?

Patient: That was before. I don't think about it now. [*looks away*] (*Engages in distancing and avoiding*)

Therapist: Can you tell me a little about what you were thinking and experiencing then? (*Asks about the patient's experience*)

Patient: Scary, uh…don't want to talk about it. I don't think about it now. (*Focusing on persecutory delusion increases the patient's anxiety.*)

Therapist: OK, Mr. Green, I won't ask you about the details. So, now it's not on your mind. You said it was before. Before when? I didn't understand what you meant. (*Moves away from past experience; asks for clarification of the patient's statement*)

Patient: You know, when I went on the pills for depression. It got better.

Therapist: Ah, so you don't have those scary thoughts so much since you started taking the medication? It's good you're taking it! (*Clarifies, connecting medication and relief from delusional thinking; adds praise*)

Patient: Yeah. That's true.

Therapist: So, let me clarify: the medication you're taking seems to have a good impact on scary thoughts and experiences. Is that accurate?

Patient: That's true. [*eye contact, brightens a little*]

Therapist: So I guess it's a good idea to keep taking it? (*Ties what the patient experiences as beneficial to a motivating statement for medication adherence*)

Patient: Yeah!…And I talk to people better. They don't seem so negative to me. (*Validates the therapist's position*)

Therapist: So the medication helps you communicate better, too? Does that mean you get along with people better than before?

Patient: I keep to myself pretty much. But I don't get into fights like I did. (*Is more elaborative as anxiety is reduced in situ*)

Therapist: You mean you got into physical fights?

Patient: Only one time. Mostly just yelling back at some of the people when I knew what they were up to.

Therapist: What were they up to? (*Asks for clarification*)

Patient: They were trying to make me look bad—said bad things about me from down the street. [*looks away*] Hmm, I don't think about it now. (**Starts to demonstrate increased anxiety, repeating his reflexive phrase**)

Therapist: So that's better now, too? That's good. What else is better? (**Goes along with the resistance; moves back to the present to reduce anxiety**)

Patient: My walls are quiet. I sleep better.

Therapist: How were they noisy?

Patient: The lady upstairs was making noise at night.

Therapist: What kind of noises? Like playing music too loud? Moving furniture?

Patient: No, uh, she would say ugly, ugly things to me. I couldn't sleep; I'd have to stay up.

Therapist: How would she talk to you?

Patient: I don't know—but it came from the wall.

Therapist: So you were hearing her voice telling you things you found unpleasant and you couldn't sleep? And it's better now? (**Clarifies**)

Patient: Yes, I can sleep again.

Therapist: That must have been a terrible time for you. I'm glad you're feeling better. What a relief that must be! (**Gives an empathic response based on the patient's statements**)

Patient: Uh-huh. [*smiles*]

Therapist: I'm going to summarize what you've told me the medication does for you, so we're clear I have it right. It takes away scary thoughts and experiences, takes away voices at night and helps you to sleep, and lets you get along with people better.

Patient: That's it.

Therapist: Sounds like good medicine!

Patient: It works.

Therapist: So can we get back to that illness that gave you the scary thoughts and experiences like voices, that kept you up and made it hard to get along with people? (**Again "shows the map"**)

Patient: OK.

Therapist: The medicine you are taking treats those symptoms of a disorder called schizophrenia—and, as we've just talked about, treats them pretty well: you're feeling a lot better than before.

Patient: I don't have that! My face didn't change. I don't attack people and drink their blood. My face didn't change. (**Becomes anxious and derails; reveals his delusional fears**)

Therapist: I think maybe you're confusing an idea you have about vampires that maybe you saw on TV—with schizophrenia. Vampires aren't real. Schizophrenia is, but it's a treatable mental disorder that has exactly the symptoms you've already described to me—symptoms that the medicine you take is good at controlling. You are not some kind of soulless monster. (**Reality-tests, clarifies, confronts, and reassures**)

Patient: What's going to happen to me? [*tears*]

Therapist: We have better medicines and better therapies than ever before, and I will be here and work with you so that you can improve the quality of your life.

## Family Psychoeducation

When supportive treatment is used with higher-functioning patients, environmental manipulation generally is not employed. However, with more impaired patients, the therapist can judiciously intervene in the patient's environment to support continued adaptation and reduce anxiety and stress. A clear example of this approach is family psychoeducation, in which educating the family changes the patient's environment. Teaching the family about the nature of the patient's disorder can help stabilize the family around the patient in a way that is more supportive of the patient's recovery. This stabilization is in contrast to the family's making the patient the focus of the family's disappointment, failed expectations, criticism, disbelief, and ignorance. Such family reactions are unlikely to help a patient cope better with chronic illness, and some of these family behaviors (e.g., high expressed emotion) are clearly associated with exacerbation of illness (Vaughn and Leff 1976). Indeed, short-term family intervention in families with high expressed emotion reduces relapse rates among patients with schizophrenia (Bellack and Mueser 1993).

## Personality Disorders

For most therapists, it is not the sickest patients (i.e., patients with psychotic symptoms and profound impairment of ego functioning) who are the most difficult to treat, but rather patients who are highly angry, demanding, suspicious, or dependent (Horowitz and Marmar 1985). Patients with personality disorders use pervasive, maladaptive interpersonal strategies, and their behaviors are sometimes dangerous or frightening. Therefore, these patients can provoke strong negative emotions in people—including psychiatrists, who may avoid treating patients with personality disorder (Lewis and Appleby 1988). The treatability of this class of disorders is contingent on several factors, including disorder severity; the specific diagnosis; the patient's degree of involvement with medical, social, and criminal justice systems; comorbidity; the availability of appropriately trained staff; and the state of scientific knowledge (Adshead 2001).

Clearly, persons administering supportive treatment to such patients must have adequate means or supervision to deal with inevitable countertransference issues, as discussed in Chapter 6, "The Therapeutic Relationship." Nonetheless, supportive psychotherapy is particularly suited to the treatment of most personality disorders, because this therapy focuses on increasing self-esteem and adaptive skills while developing and maintaining a strong therapeutic alliance. As described in Chapter 4, "Assessment, Case Formulation, Goal Setting, and Outcome Research," the psychiatrist must conduct an assessment of the patient that allows for a case formulation, including an explication of ego functioning, adaptive skills, object relations, and defensive operations. In certain clusters of personality disorders, patients appear to make greater use of particular groups of maladaptive defenses and defensive behaviors. For example, in the treatment of patients with avoidant personality disorder, a major focus is on getting the patient to develop skills to overcome passivity and fears of rejection. In contrast, with narcissistic personality disorder, the focus is on addressing and reducing uses of externalization and criticism. The clinician decides at what point to use more containing, anxiety-reducing supportive technique and when to use expressive technique.

It is important to identify comorbid mood and anxiety disorders. In contrast to earlier concerns that medicating patients would deprive them of the motivation for engagement in treatment, today it is recognized that judicious pharmacological treatment of comorbid depression and anxiety disorders generally acts synergistically with the personality disorder patient's attempts at learning and mastering new adaptive skills. In depressed patients, pharmacotherapy reduces Cluster C personality pathology—in particular, harm avoidance, which is associated with poor social function (Hellerstein et al. 2000; Kool et al. 2003; Peselow et al. 1994). When patients are less anxious or less depressed, they are more willing to explore new strategies and may be better able to do so. (See Chapter 4 for an evaluation of a patient with major depressive disorder.)

In a review of the effectiveness of psychotherapies for personality disorder, J.C. Perry and colleagues (1999) found that all studies of active psychotherapies reported positive outcomes at termination and follow-up. In addition, patients receiving treatment have an accelerated rate of recovery from personality disorders, compared with the natural course of the disorders. Bateman and Fonagy (2000) also conducted a systematic review of the evidence for efficacy of psychotherapy in personality disorders. Although psychotherapy was found to be effective, the evidence did not indicate that one form of treatment is superior to another. However, effective treatments were found to have several factors in common, including encouragement of a strong relationship between patient and therapist that would allow the therapist to take an active rather than passive stance.

Rosenthal and colleagues (1999) demonstrated lasting change in interpersonal functioning among patients with Cluster C personality disorders who were treated with 40 sessions of manual-based supportive psychotherapy. In addition, in patients with major depression and personality disorders (especially Cluster C personality disorders), short-term (16-session) supportive psychotherapy in combination with antidepressant treatment reduces personality pathology, compared with antidepressant treatment alone (Kool et al. 2003). Patients with problems of hostile dominance, such as patients with antisocial personality disorder, tend to receive less demonstrable benefit from supportive psychotherapy than patients with other personality disorders (Kool et al. 2003; Woody et al. 1985). However, when there is comorbid depression, patients with antisocial personality disorder may do well. It has been hypothesized that the benefit is related to the patients' having some capacity to form a therapeutic alliance (Gerstley et al. 1989).

It has been posited that in supportive psychotherapy, when transference interpretation does not occur, the character-transforming factor is the patient's capacity to form an identification with the more benign, accepting attitude of the therapist (Appelbaum and Levy 2002; Pinsker et al. 1991). For example, patients with borderline personality disorder typically must contend with what in structural terms can be modeled as a rigid, archaic, and punitive superego. Identification with the therapist may allow the patient to be more tolerant of hateful and shameful aspects of the self.

Holmes (1995) reported on borderline patients' use of the commitment, concern, and attention of supportive technique during analytic treatment and suggested that the development of secure attachments fostered more autonomous functioning. By discouraging destructive behaviors, the therapist models more appropriate behavior and demonstrates strength and concern for the patient (Appelbaum and Levy 2002). As injurious behaviors diminish, the patient can identify with the reflective function of the therapist.

Appelbaum and Levy (2002) pointed out that the supportive therapist strives to establish in the patient an arousal level optimal for learning, fostering a sense of self, and appreciating the consequences of behavior. These factors are not unlike those in successful parenting, as Misch (2000) noted, and help to address ego and adaptive dysfunction in patients with borderline personality disorder. With such patients, the therapist works to create a sense of safety in order to reduce maladaptive defenses, which are typically linked to fears of annihilation, abandonment, and humiliation. Creating a sense of safety can help the patient begin to develop a more integrated sense of self and other in the context of reduced anxiety. Nevertheless, this sense of safety must be created without fostering regression, which can escalate those behaviors that the therapist is trying to address and reduce. Maladaptive or immature defenses such as regression, denial, or projection are not supported. As in much of supportive psychotherapy, there is the continuing balance of supportive and expressive technique.

An advance in the treatment of borderline personality disorder was the development of dialectical behavior therapy (DBT), which initially focused on reducing parasuicidal behavior (Linehan 1993; Linehan et al. 1994). Although this practical, multicomponent approach to therapy with borderline patients has been presented as an evolution of cognitive-behavioral therapy, certain of the main components of the treatment are decidedly supportive, in that they directly address ego function and adaptive skills. The open and explicit collaboration between patient and therapist on here-and-now issues in DBT is consistent with the style of supportive treatment. In particular, the use of mindfulness exercises is a direct measure that addresses both ego functioning and adaptive skill, in teaching patients to develop intrapsychic distance from overwhelming emotional distress. In addition, DBT makes liberal use of slogans and sayings that reframe patients' isolated experience into shared experiential wisdom and that serve as feedback for validating both subjective states and real responsibility (Palmer 2002).

## Substance Use Disorders

Substance use disorders are among the most common mental disorders in the population (Regier et al. 1990). Traditionally, most psychiatry residents did not treat patients presenting with substance use disorders unless the patients presented with co-occurring psychiatric disorders (see "Co-occurring Mental Illness and Substance Use Disorders" later in this chapter). Generally, residents learned about withdrawal syndromes and detoxification on inpatient psychiatric units that admitted patients with psychiatric disorders or substance-induced mental disorders. Currently, residency training in psychiatry involves at least 1 month of full-time clinical work with patients who have substance use disorders, and thus, residents must learn about basic psychotherapeutic and medication management of these patients. There are few effective pharmacotherapies for substance use disorders, and those therapies work best in the context of psychosocial treatment. Therefore, psychotherapy is an important intervention for substance use disorders. Medications approved for use in substance use disorders are maintenance medications for opioid dependence—such as methadone and buprenorphine (Fudala et al. 2003; Kleber 2003)—or for alcohol dependence—either aversive medications such as disulfiram (Fuller et al. 1986) or craving reducers such as naltrexone (O'Malley et al. 1992; Volpicelli et al. 1992).

In the past, individual expressive treatments were the standard intervention for substance use disorders. Over time, it became clear that use of uncovering psychotherapy as a sole mode of treatment for substance use disorders was generally not effective. Other treatment approaches, such as group therapies, pharmacotherapies (e.g., methadone maintenance), and therapeutic communities, became mainstays of addiction treatment. Rounsaville and Carroll (1998) underscored the rationale for supportive psychotherapy when they described the reasons that expressive treatments, when offered as the sole ambulatory treatment, are not well suited to the needs of patients with substance use disorders. In expressive treatments, there is a lack of focus on symptom control and development of coping skills. Patients drop out frequently because of a lack a focus on the patient's presenting problem and because patients find the therapist's neutral, abstaining stance anxiety provoking. Today, we understand that interpretations of addictive behaviors are not sufficient to stop the addictive process and that increasing the patient's anxiety early in the treatment of a substance use disorder is likely to trigger a relapse. So a more uncovering type of treatment should be embarked on only when the patient has established a concrete method for maintaining abstinence or is being treated within a protected environment (Brill 1977; Rosenthal and Westreich 1999).

To conduct psychotherapy with substance-abusing patients, the therapist must understand the psychopharmacology of commonly abused classes of drugs, typical presentations of intoxication and withdrawal, and the natural course of drug effects. It is also necessary to become familiar with common or street knowledge about the drugs, including slang names and prices (Rounsaville and Carroll 1998). A good working knowledge of the drugs of abuse and the lifestyle of the drug-abusing patient can help the therapist begin to build a therapeutic alliance with the patient.

Supportive psychotherapy with substance use disorder patients focuses on helping the patient to develop effective coping strategies to control or reduce substance use and stay engaged in treatment. Other important aspects are developing and maintaining a strong therapeutic alliance and helping the patient to both reduce and learn to manage anxiety and dysphoria in order to minimize the risk of relapse. Because supportive psychotherapy offers a broad and flexible foundation for interventions with patients, work with addicted patients typically includes use of newer, more evidence-based strategies, such as motivational interviewing, relapse prevention, and psychoeducation. General supportive principles are maintained during the course of addiction treatment, even as patient and therapist embark on particular cognitive and behavioral work such as building cognitive skills. With substance use disorders, individual supportive psychotherapy is often augmented and supported by the patient's engagement in 12-step programs, group therapies for substance use disorders, and other recovery-oriented therapeutic activities.

## Motivational Interviewing

If an individual is not interested in reducing or stopping the use of substances when he or she meets the criteria for a substance use disorder, the person may have a diagnosis, but he or she is not yet a patient. People who come into treatment for substance use disorders typically have spent months to years without severe consequences and have experienced the drug use as fun or beneficial. People generally show up for substance abuse treatment only when the consequences of their drug use have become threatening to their relationships, employment, health, freedom, or life. At that time, most people bring with them beliefs about their drug use that were constructed when their use appeared to be free of severe negative consequences. In addition, a common belief from that time is that drugs play an essential role in the individual's ability to cope (Rounsaville and Carroll 1998). It is clear in this context that unless the patient sees the substance abuse as a problem and can conceptualize getting along without drug use, it is going to be difficult to set appropriate treatment goals.

Rollnick and Miller (1995) described motivational interviewing as a directive, patient-centered intervention that helps patients to explore and resolve their ambivalence about changing. The main principles of motivational interviewing include understanding the patient's view accurately, avoiding or de-escalating resistance, and increasing the patient's self-efficacy and perception of the discrepancy between actual and ideal behavior (Miller and Rollnick 1991). Motivational interviewing is explicitly empathic and does not involve a coercive therapist position with respect to the patient's actions about reducing or stopping substance use; the patient might experience such a position as demeaning and damaging to self-esteem. A premise of motivational interviewing is that patients can decide to make changes based on their own shifts in motivation. The techniques of motivational interviewing include listening reflectively and eliciting motivational statements from patients, examining both sides of patients' ambivalence, and reducing resistance by monitoring patient readiness and not pushing for change prematurely (Miller and Rollnick 1991). When the patient experiences that the negative consequences of substance use outweigh the positives ones, the so-called decisional balance is tipped in favor of engagement in treatment.

There is substantial evidence that motivational interviewing is an effective intervention for substance use disorders—especially with regard to promoting entry into and engagement in more-intensive substance abuse treatment—even when the technique is used by clinicians who are not substance abuse treatment specialists (Dunn et al. 2001). Therefore, motivational interviewing is a mainstay of supportive treatment of substance use disorders.

## Adaptive Skills and Relapse Prevention

The main content of supportive treatment of substance use disorders is the work of achieving and maintaining abstinence from substances of abuse. Patients must learn new strategies that assist them in coping with craving states, negative emotions, general stress, and cues in the environment that serve as high-risk triggers for substance use. Long ago, the proponents of Alcoholic Anonymous identified exposure to the "people, places, and things" associated with alcohol use as a primer to relapse. It is said that stopping the use of drugs is relatively easy—remaining drug free is the hard part. The specific adaptive skills that must be learned in addiction recovery are 1) identifying high-risk situations and cues, 2) anticipating exposure to these situations and cues, and 3) developing alternative strategies for coping when exposed to these situations.

Relapse prevention is a formal set of cognitive-behavioral approaches to maintaining abstinence that are easily woven into supportive treatment. In relapse prevention, a systematic effort is made to identify the patient's specific relapse triggers and to devise and have the patient practice alternative behaviors and coping skills to deal with these triggers, such as refusal skills for when the patient is offered the target substance (Marlatt and Gordon 1985). However, identification of risky situations and development of coping skills to address these situations can also be done in a less structured fashion in supportive and supportive-expressive psychotherapy (Luborsky 1984). In any case, anticipatory guidance, encouragement, and reassurance are key supportive techniques that are used when identifying and rehearsing skills to cope with an expected situation. The therapist works to establish achievable intermediate goals, to reduce the risk of failure and of further damage to the patient's self-esteem. When the patient brings in a report that he or she has successfully negotiated some element of a high-risk situation, praise related to the patient's goals is meaningful and reinforces the improvement in adaptive skills. The patient should have already experienced some increase in self-esteem through an experience of competence in achieving a life skill. If the patient tries and does not succeed, some praise is indicated, because the patient tried to implement the adaptive skill. The therapist encourages the patient to try the skill again, and reassures him about doing so, after they do some problem solving. Thus, progress in executing new skills may be incremental, and the therapist offers measured but increasingly intense praise and positive feedback for each successive goal met.

Because a dysphoric mood is the most frequently reported antecedent of relapse, it is equally important that the supportive treatment of substance use disorders focus on building adaptive skills for coping with negative or painful mood states (Marlatt and Gordon 1980). Substance-abusing individuals often have a difficult time differentiating mood states into specific affects, in part perhaps because they use the drugs to self-medicate dysphoria, rather than developing psychological means to cope with the painful affects (Keller et al. 1995; Khantzian 1985). So it is important to work with substance use disorder patients to help them begin to reduce alexithymia in distinguishing one feeling from another. As Misch (2000) described, the ability to identify and label feelings makes it easier to reflect on them and communicate about them to others. If the patient cannot notice and discriminate feelings, he or she cannot make clear connections between those feelings and the thoughts, behaviors, or events linked to drug use. For example, if patients cannot recognize when they are irritable and sad, they will not be able to connect either state to the automatic thoughts that they generate in response, such as "I'm feeling irritated, so I must get a bottle." The ability to label feelings is essential for developing appropriate adaptive skills to manage painful affects. As patients begin to identify these feelings, they experience—in spite of increased awareness of negative affect—an increase in self-esteem that comes from mastery of the internal environment. The affects begin to be reframed as useful tools in identifying risky states that set patients up for relapse.

## Psychoeducation

In the area of substance use disorders, education efforts focus on teaching patients about different classes of abused drugs, psychological and physical effects of drugs, dangers of chronic abuse, the fact that drugs may be used to self-medicate, and a disease model of addiction. Most cultures implicitly or explicitly operate out of a moral model of substance abuse and addiction, which attributes the irresponsible or criminal behavior of the addicted individual to his or her bad character. In contrast, the unitary disease concept of addiction, variously attributed to Alcoholics

Anonymous (1976) or Jellinek (1952), stresses that addiction is a chronic, relapsing, and progressive illness. Further, the advocates of the "disease concept" thought it was a mistake to think of alcoholism as a symptom of another disorder, such that if an underlying conflict were resolved in expressive treatment, the patient would stop drinking (Rosenthal and Westreich 1999). Jellinek's approach to alcoholism was not actually so reductionistic; he in fact described several typologies, which differed regarding onset, severity, pattern, and chronicity of use. Nonetheless, the psychotherapeutic utility of this heuristic approach is that it increases self-esteem by offering the patient a diagnosis rather than blame, helps the patient cope better with shame (given that most patients presume that the moral model explains their own behavior), and offers another frame in which to foster a therapeutic alliance.

The following dialogue illustrates the use of psychoeducation with a substance-abusing patient:

> Patient: I can't stop it…the crack. I got thrown out of the house…no job, no girl, no money, no nothing…'cept the crack. I've blown up my life. [*sighs, looks at therapist*] Why bother? Maybe they're right, and I'm no good. [*looks down, shakes head, tears*] No good, just no good… (***Attributes his drug-related losses and maladaptive behavior to being a bad person***)
>
> Therapist: I know the pain you're feeling makes you want to just blame yourself. And you've got a lot of reasons to feel bad right now. But can I ask you to consider something about your intentions for a moment? It's important, but it will require a bit of reflection. (***Empathically turns the patient's focus away from self-blame to cognition***)
>
> Patient: OK.
>
> Therapist: If you really knew before you started that the result of your using crack would be what your life is like right now and how you feel now, would you have done it anyway? (***Clarifies***)
>
> Patient: Nah, don't think so. No, no way! [angry] (***Takes rational position***)
>
> Therapist: So, I want you to know that the situation you are in now is very predictable. When people get addicted to crack, this is what happens to them. Addiction is like a runaway train. If you get on board, you go where it takes you, not where you think you want to go. (***Generalizes to others who have the same well-described problem; offers teaching metaphor***)
>
> Patient: Yeah, but I'm the one who started it, and I keep doing it—I don't stop. Something's wrong with me! I must be stupid, stupid! (***Retreats to moral-model explanation; holds on to denial of loss of control***)
>
> Therapist: Well, I guess blaming yourself still gives you some sense that it's under your control and OK, when it's clearly not! If you are stu-

pid, then that's a way to explain the situation, but you are not stupid. You already told me that you wouldn't purposely choose to be in this situation and that you can't stop. That's why we talk about it as a disease. The loss of control comes with the territory; it's part of the disease. People try to control it, and it somehow always gets away from them. The drug is powerful in that way. Let me show you the diagnostic criteria for substance dependence. Loss of control is in there as a major symptom. [*Opens DSM-IV-TR to criteria for substance dependence and reads criterion 3, about use of a greater quantity or longer use than intended, and criterion 4, about unsuccessful efforts to cut down or control use*] (**Confronts denial, which is maladaptive for this patient; offers a different explanation; uses props to concretize the ideas**)

Patient: So many times I tried to only do some, but I spent everything I had. [*sad*]

Therapist: So, yes, you were responsible for trying the drug initially and thinking you could get away with it. But what's wrong with you now is that you have a real disorder. You know drinking runs in families—the risk is inherited—and drug problems are similar. (**Supports patient's understanding with clarification and new knowledge**)

Patient: My dad was alcoholic. So was my uncle, and I think maybe it killed him. (**Confirms the understanding that his problems are more than just about willpower**)

Therapist: In many ways, this is not your fault, but there is something you can do. Now maybe you can see it is your responsibility to work with me—to help you fight this bad disease. (**Sides with the patient against the disease; supports the need for collaboration**)

Patient: It feels like it's impossible. Can I really get help with this? (**Elicits reassurance**)

Therapist: The good news is that although it's a lot of work, addiction is treatable like other chronic illnesses. We don't have a cure yet for diabetes and high blood pressure, but people can recover from the illness being out of control and have better lives.

# Co-occurring Mental Illness and Substance Use Disorders

About half the population with severe mental disorders is affected by substance abuse or dependence (Regier et al. 1990). In clinical samples of psychiatric patients, there are often higher rates of alcohol use disorders and other substance use disorders (Fernandez-Pol et al. 1988; Fischer et al. 1975; Galanter et al. 1988; Richard et al. 1985). Kessler et al. (1994) found, in the National Comorbidity Survey, that of the population who had psychosis or mania or needed hospitalization for a mental disorder in a 12-month period, almost 90% met the criteria for three or more lifetime alcohol or drug use disorders or mental disorders.

It is well established that co-occurrence of mental illness and substance use disorders has a negative effect on the trajectory of and recovery from both disorders (Rosenthal and Westreich 1999). Patients with substance use disorders and schizophrenia are also well described as being difficult to engage in treatment, so supportive psychotherapy, with its focus on building and maintaining a therapeutic alliance, is indicated for this population (Carey et al. 1996; Lehman et al. 1993). Supportive treatment for those with both disorders integrates the techniques that are useful for each problem, as delineated in "Severe Mental Illness" and "Substance Use Disorders" earlier in this chapter. Improving adaptive skills by increasing competence in basic conversational and recreational skills, using medication and symptom management, and using relapse prevention for negotiating situations likely to trigger relapse to substance abuse are all generally needed to treat co-occurring substance use disorders and mental illness. Implementing these interventions has a beneficial effect on treatment retention and substance use in patients with psychotic illness and substance use disorders (Ho et al. 1999). Multiple studies have shown that psychosocial treatment that integrates psychiatric and addiction treatment components leads to better retention and better outcome among patients with severe mental illness and substance use disorders (Drake et al. 2001; Hellerstein et al. 1995).

Additional factors that work in concert with individual supportive treatment are support for patient involvement in 12-step programs (especially programs that are less likely to reduce self-esteem, such as "double trouble" or "dual recovery" groups) and family psychoeducation. Support for access to concrete services, socialization, recreation, and other opportunities can serve, in addition to praise, as positive reinforcement for attendance and may support the development of a therapeutic alliance and the engagement of patients in treatment (Rosenthal et al. 2000).

## Psychoeducation

In the context of supportive treatment, patients with substance use disorders and mental illness should be given information about both classes of disorders. Like other supportive techniques, psychoeducation must be formulated in the context of the therapist's appraisal of the patient's capacity to make use of the information in a way that supports ego function or adaptive skills. For example, when a patient with a severe mental illness learns that he or she has another chronic illness such as substance dependence, this knowledge can become a factor in his or her demoralization (Rosenthal and Westreich 1999). As in supportive treatment of patients without substance disorders, the therapist also teaches about the mental illness: its symptoms, treatment, and natural history. Patients are encouraged to discuss their own symptoms and their own history of treatment responsiveness and to attempt to understand what role their substance abuse may have played in either relieving or exacerbating psychotic, mood, and anxiety symptoms.

Most patients with co-occurring substance use disorders and severe mental disorders who come into contact with treatment systems are not interested in stopping use of substances and are not motivated to stop use. With these patients, motivational interviewing techniques can be useful within the context of supportive psychotherapy (Ziedonis and Fisher 1996; Ziedonis and Trudeau 1997). The process of recovery in patients with comorbid substance use disorders and mental disorders is not linear, and exacerbation of both disorders is episodic. Patients may cycle repeatedly through different phases of treatment—engagement, active treatment, maintenance, relapse, and then reengagement. When patients come back into contact with treating clinicians after a relapse, they may be in an earlier motivational stage; they may even be in denial that a substance abuse problem exists (Prochaska and DiClemente 1984). Motivational techniques, which are traditionally used at the beginning of therapy to engage substance use disorder patients in treatment, are thus used as a continuing component of supportive treatment in patients with co-occurring substance use disorders and severe mental illness. This approach is needed because patients cycle between motivational levels, with the various flare-ups of substance use disorders and other mental illness over time (Rosenthal and Westreich 1999). For patients with dual diagnoses, the time frame of recovery from substance use disorders is longer than that for patients without comorbid severe mental disorders. However, if the patient remains in treatment, reduction in severity of both disorders is a realistic prospect (Drake et al. 1993; Hellerstein et al. 1995).

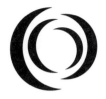

# 9

# Evaluating Competence

The Accreditation Council for Graduate Medical Education (ACGME) defined six areas of competence for medical trainees: 1) patient care, 2) medical knowledge, 3) practice-based learning and improvement, 4) interpersonal and communication skills, 5) professionalism, and 6) systems-based practice (ACGME Outcomes Project 2000). Outlining and describing areas of competence are within our grasp at the present time. However, defining, evaluating, and measuring competence of trainees is another matter. Development of measurement tools and their application to specific areas of competence is under way but still in an early stage. The ACGME suggested a dozen methods of measuring competence. These methods, which the ACGME labeled "the Toolbox," include various types of written, oral, and clinical examinations; a combined assessment approach of patient, family, supervisors, and others; record reviews; portfolios and case logs; simulations, models, and use of standardized patients; and evaluation of live or recorded performance. The Residency Review Committee for Psychiatry chose five areas of psychotherapy in which residents in psychiatry must be certified as competent by their training programs. In this chapter, we outline our approach to evaluating competence of psychiatry trainees in one of these psychotherapies—namely, supportive psychotherapy.

A major issue to be addressed is the definition of *competence*. An acceptable definition of *competent* is "having requisite or adequate ability or qualities" (*Merriam-Webster's Collegiate Dictionary*, 11th edition). Epstein and Hundert (2002) defined professional competence as "the habitual and judicious use of communication, knowledge, technical skills, clinical reasoning, emotions, values and reflection in daily practice for the benefit of the individual and community being served" (p. 226). In assessments of trainees, one should look for competence, not a high level of expertise (Manring et al. 2003).

When assessing a resident's competence, it is necessary to define what will be assessed and the method or methods of assessment. In addition, the evaluation process should be educational and promote resident learning. Professional competence can be conceptualized as a continuum of levels of ability or skill, from beginner to competent to expert. A trainee would be expected to be competent and thus be at the middle of this continuum.

## Psychotherapy Supervision

Assessment of residents' competence in psychotherapy is an ongoing process in many residency programs. In the main, evaluations of residents are performed by clinical supervisors during the process of psychotherapy supervision and are formally discussed with the residents one or more times a year.

Clinical supervision, as well as more formal seminars and classroom teaching, has long been a part of psychotherapy training. Seminars and classroom approaches generally consist of reading courses, in which psychotherapy theory and practice are taught, and clinical case seminars, which focus on evaluation, case formulation, diagnosis, and ongoing psychotherapy. Many training programs in psychiatry have established traditions of intensive individual supervision of residents, particularly in long-term expressive (exploratory) psychotherapy. The process of supervision may vary from one program to another but generally involves the following:

1. Presentation of the case by the resident
2. Discussion of the diagnosis, the case formulation, goals, and the treatment plan
3. Ongoing summary of sessions by the resident, using an informal recall-and-summary approach, process notes, videotapes, or a combination of these approaches
4. Discussion of the psychotherapy process, including resistance, dysfunctional thinking, defenses, affect, and therapist interventions, as well as dynamics, genetics, psychological structure, cognitive-behavioral issues, and the therapeutic relationship (transference, countertransference, and the therapeutic alliance)

The supervisor has traditionally evaluated the resident's work by noting how well the resident performs the tasks just listed, as well as assessing other areas such as the ability to listen and relate to the patient in an empathic manner. The evaluation process by the supervisor is ongoing, but formal evaluations are generally performed once or twice a year or more. The formal evaluations are based on material discussed by the trainee through the use of process notes. Traditionally, the entire process has been somewhat informal and rarely standardized. In this chapter, we propose a standardized evaluation approach, one based on the use of videotapes during an ongoing course of psychotherapy.

## Focus of Assessment

Assessment of competence in supportive psychotherapy should be evaluated within the broader context of general psychotherapy. The assessment should encompass skills of, attitudes toward, and knowledge about general psychotherapy and the more specific approach of supportive psychotherapy. General psychotherapy skills were described by the American Association of Directors of Psychiatric Residency Training (AADPRT) Psychotherapy Task Force (2000) and include establishing and maintaining boundaries and the therapeutic alliance, listening, addressing emotions, understanding, using supervision, dealing with resistances and defenses, and applying intervention techniques. Beitman and Yue (1999) described a similar set of skills, which they called core psychotherapy skills and which include other skills such as identifying patterns and implementing strategies for change. The AADPRT Psychotherapy Task Force also developed psychotherapy competencies for the five psychotherapies mandated by the Residency Review Committee for Psychiatry, including supportive psychotherapy. See Table 9–1 for a complete list of the AADPRT competencies for supportive psychotherapy (AADPRT 2003).

The supportive psychotherapy competencies are divided into skills of, attitudes toward, and knowledge about supportive therapy. The skills section contains 15 items, including the ability to maintain a therapeutic alliance, the ability to use appropriate interventions, and the ability to establish treatment goals. The attitudes section includes an empathic, respectful, nonjudgmental approach and sensitivity to sociocultural, socioeconomic, and educational issues. The knowledge category encompasses knowledge about objectives, the patient–therapist relationship, and indications and contraindications for supportive therapy.

| **Table 9–1.** | American Association of Directors of Psychiatric Residency Training competencies for supportive psychotherapy |
|---|---|

**Knowledge**

1. The resident will demonstrate knowledge that the principal objectives of supportive therapy are to maintain or improve the patient's self-esteem, minimize or prevent recurrence of symptoms, and maximize the patient's adaptive capacities.
2. The resident will demonstrate understanding that the practice of supportive therapy is commonly used in many therapeutic encounters.
3. The resident will demonstrate knowledge that the patient–therapist relationship is of paramount importance.
4. The resident will demonstrate knowledge of indications and contraindications for supportive therapy.
5. The resident will demonstrate understanding that continued education in supportive therapy is necessary for further skill development.

**Skills**

1. The resident will be able to establish and maintain a therapeutic alliance.
2. The resident will be able to establish treatment goals.
3. The resident will be able to interact in a direct and nonthreatening manner.
4. The resident will be able to be responsive to the patient and give feedback and advice when appropriate.
5. The resident will demonstrate the ability to understand the patient as a unique individual within his or her family and sociocultural community.
6. The resident will be able to determine which interventions are in the best interest of the patient and will exercise caution about basing interventions on his or her own beliefs and values.
7. The resident will be able to recognize and identify affects in the patient and himself or herself.
8. The resident will be able to confront in a collaborative manner behaviors that are dangerous or damaging to the patient.
9. The resident will be able to provide reassurance to reduce symptoms, improve morale and adaptation, and prevent relapse.
10. The resident will be able to support, promote, and recognize the patient's ability to achieve goals that will promote his or her well-being.
11. The resident will be able to provide strategies to manage problems with affect regulation, thoughts disorders, and impaired reality-testing.
12. The resident will be able to provide education and advice about the patient's psychiatric condition, treatment, and adaptation while being sensitive to specific community systems of care and sociocultural issues.
13. The resident will be able to demonstrate that in the care of patients with chronic disorders, attention should be directed to adaptive skills, relationships, morale, and potential sources of anxiety or worry.
14. The resident will be able to assist the patient in developing skills for self-assessment.

---

**Table 9–1.** American Association of Directors of Psychiatric
Residency Training competencies for supportive
psychotherapy *(continued)*

---

15. The resident will be able to seek appropriate consultation and/or referral for specialized treatment.

**Attitudes**
1. The resident will be empathic, respectful, curious, open, nonjudgmental, collaborative, and able to tolerate ambiguity and display confidence in the efficacy of supportive therapy.
2. The resident will be sensitive to sociocultural, socioeconomic, and educational issues that arise in the therapeutic relationship.
3. The resident will be open to audiotaping, videotaping, or direct observation of treatment sessions.

---

*Source.*  American Association of Directors of Psychiatry Residency Training 2001.

# Method of Assessment

Assessment of a trainee's competence in supportive psychotherapy can be accomplished using a number of different methodologies, including administration of written and/or oral examinations that test the resident's knowledge base, use of simulated patients reading from standardized scripts, the request that the resident respond to a patient vignette using a supportive approach, and a supervisor's evaluation of a resident performing supportive psychotherapy. We have found that supervisor evaluations of ongoing, videotaped psychotherapy sessions are the best method of teaching and evaluating residents. Videotaped sessions enable the supervisor or resident evaluator to observe the conduct of psychotherapy directly. The more traditional method of summarizing a session or working from process notes is less likely to convey what actually took place in a psychotherapy session, even under the best of circumstances. The availability of video recordings opens the process of psychotherapy to an outside observer and makes evaluation of therapy more objective.

Evaluation of videotaped supportive psychotherapy sessions should begin with the resident's assessment of the patient and should continue for the entire psychotherapy. Each supervision session should begin with a brief summary by the resident, followed by a review of the videotape. It is highly unlikely that an entire videotape can be reviewed in a supervisory hour, so the supervisor and resident must decide which segments to review. The choice of videotaped segments for viewing can be based on the resident's summary, which may point to areas of difficulty or significance. A formal written evaluation of the resident by the supervisor should be completed at least twice a year. This evaluation should be educative and be based on the supervisory work preceding the formal evaluation. The supervisor should provide the resident with verbal feedback on a regular basis.

Having trainees view tapes of psychotherapy sessions conducted by others essentially replaces a supervisory experience and can be used to assess evaluation of knowledge, which cannot always be equated with skill. This procedure allows for discussion of techniques and of the broad range of possible therapeutic interventions.

## Assessment Instrument

The AADPRT supportive therapy competencies provide the basis for development of a rating form to be used as a measure of resident's competence in supportive psychotherapy. The proposed form (Figure 9–1) does not include all the items on the AADPRT list of competencies, because it would not be practical or reasonable for training programs to use lengthy evaluation forms for five different psychotherapies. In addition, some items were modified or combined with other items from the supportive therapy and general psychotherapy competencies.

The evaluation form covers three areas: knowledge, skills, and attitudes. For example, the first item in the knowledge and attitudes section is the following: "The resident demonstrates knowledge that the principal objectives of supportive therapy are to maintain or improve the patient's self-esteem, ameliorate or prevent recurrence of symptoms, improve psychological or ego functioning, and enhance adaptive capacities." The rating is on a Likert scale of 0–5 (0=can't say, 1=unsatisfactory, 2=approaching competence, 3=competent, 4=competent plus, 5=expert). In the skills section, item 1 is the following: "The resident is able to establish and maintain a positive therapeutic alliance and interact with the patient in an empathic, respectful, direct, responsive, nonthreatening manner." An item taken from general psychotherapy competencies, placed in the knowledge and attitudes section (item 5), is worded thus: "The resident understands that appropriate boundaries (e.g., time, outside agencies and relationships, confidentiality, and professional attitude) must be established and maintained."

The advantages of this evaluation form are that it can be scored and that it also includes space for the supervisor's comments. The final score is calculated by dividing the number of questions answered from 1 to 5 into the total score. An average score of 3 or better suggests that the resident has demonstrated competence in supportive therapy. In addition,

## Resident Evaluation for Competence in Supportive Psychotherapy

Resident _____ Supervisor_____

Date_____ Period _____

*Instructions: Please evaluate the resident's performance on the following items by circling the appropriate number.*

| Can't say | Unsatisfactory | Approaching competence | Competent | Competent plus | Expert |
|-----------|----------------|------------------------|-----------|----------------|--------|
| 0 | 1 | 2 | 3 | 4 | 5 |

### Knowledge and attitudes

1. The resident demonstrates knowledge that the principal objectives of supportive therapy are to maintain or improve the patient's self-esteem, ameliorate or prevent recurrence of symptoms, improve psychological or ego functioning, and enhance adaptive capacities.
2. The resident understands that supportive therapy is dynamically based and is part of a continuum ranging from supportive to expressive therapy.
3. The resident demonstrates knowledge that the patient–therapist relationship is of paramount importance and is not addressed unless it is negative.
4. The resident demonstrates knowledge of indications and contraindications for supportive psychotherapy.
5. The resident understands that appropriate boundaries (e.g., time, outside agencies and relationships, confidentiality, and professional attitude) must be established and maintained.

### Skills

1. The resident is able to establish and maintain a positive therapeutic alliance and interact with the patient in an empathic, respectful, direct, responsive, nonthreatening manner.
2. The resident relates to the patient in a conversational manner (i.e., does not interrogate or engage in passive listening).
3. The resident is able to establish realistic and appropriate treatment goals.
4. The resident uses supportive therapy interventions (clarification, confrontation, interpretation, advice, reassurance, encouragement, praise, rationalization, reframing) in an appropriate and timely manner.
5. The resident is able to respect and strengthen adaptive defenses, distinguish between adaptive and maladaptive defenses, and work to minimize anxiety in an appropriate and timely manner.
6. The resident provides education about the patient's psychiatric condition and medication and, if necessary, about community systems of care and ancillary treatments.
7. The resident focuses on the patient's present-day life, while not ignoring the past, and consistently works at improving self-esteem, promoting adaptation and ego functions, and ameliorating symptoms.

*Supervisor's comments (include comments on overall performance, strengths, areas needing further work, and the ability to work in and use supervision):*

_____

_____

_____

*Resident's signature (this evaluation was discussed with me)*

_____

*Supervisor's signature*

**Figure 9–1.** Supportive psychotherapy evaluation form.

the supervisor should also write some overall comments about the resident, including the resident's strengths and overall performance, areas needing further work, and the resident's ability to work in and use supervision. The supervisor should discuss the evaluation with the resident in a way that is supportive and promotes the resident's education.

To standardize the evaluation of competence in supportive therapy, it would be important to have conferences with the supportive psychotherapy supervisors to discuss the supervisory and evaluation process. One method of achieving reliability would be to have groups of supervisors rate supportive psychotherapy videotapes and then discuss their ratings. Discussions would be directed at reaching a consensus in the evaluation ratings. This approach has been used in psychotherapy research to measure therapist adherence to manual-based forms of psychotherapy (Waltz et al. 1993).

A number of questions have been raised about the feasibility of using videotaped recordings of psychotherapy for supervision. Difficulties cited include the cost and maintenance of the equipment and the ability of residents to operate the recording equipment. The cost of video equipment has decreased during the past decade, enabling many training programs to offer videotaping to residents. At the same time, video equipment has become easy to operate, and residents are able to make good recordings. Therefore, it seems feasible for residency programs to provide video equipment for residency training in psychotherapy.

In the event that video equipment cannot be provided by the institution, it would not be unreasonable to require each trainee to provide his or her own camera. After all, the training program does not provide each resident with textbooks. The essential feature of videorecording is not a high-quality picture but understandable audio on a tape that runs without attention for the entire session.

Some residency programs may not be ready to begin with evaluations involving video. The evaluation form presented in this chapter can be used to evaluate a trainee reporting on psychotherapy sessions from process notes. Another approach would be to present a videotape or written material from a supportive therapy session and ask the resident questions about the treatment plan, case formulation, goals, technique, alliance, and so on. In addition, the resident could be asked to respond to the patient's complaints using a supportive psychotherapy approach.

## Summary

This chapter provides an overview of current efforts to evaluate the competence of residents engaged in various clinical tasks. We have presented a preliminary approach to evaluating psychiatry residents in supportive psychotherapy, an approach involving adaptation of the AADPRT list of supportive therapy competencies into an evaluation form. However, the process of evaluating competence is in an early phase of development and will require a great deal of reflection, planning, and study to achieve reliable and valid measurement systems.

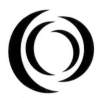

# References

Accreditation Council for Graduate Medical Education (ACGME) Outcomes Project: Toolbox of Assessment Methods, Version 1.1. September 2000. Available at: http://www.acgme.org/Outcome/assess/Toolbox.pdf. Accessed January 6, 2004.

Adshead G: Murmurs of discontent: treatment and treatability of personality disorder. Advances in Psychiatric Treatment 7:407–417, 2001

Aguilera DC, Messick J, Farrel LM: Crisis Intervention. St. Louis, MO, Mosby, 1970

Alcoholics Anonymous: The Story of How Many Thousands of Men and Women Have Recovered From Alcoholism, 3rd Edition. New York, Alcoholics Anonymous World Service, 1976, p 12

Alexander F, French TM: Psychoanalytic Psychotherapy. New York, Ronald Press, 1946

Alstrom JE, Nordlund CL, Persson G, et al: Effects of four treatment methods on social phobia patients not suitable for insight-oriented psychotherapy. Acta Psychiatr Scand 70:1–17, 1984

Alter CL: Palliative and supportive care of patients with pancreatic cancer. Semin Oncol 23:229–240, 1996

American Association of Directors of Psychiatric Residency Training (AADPRT): AADPRT supportive therapy competencies. Farmington, CT, American Association of Directors of Psychiatric Residency Training, 2001. Available at: http://www.aadprt.org/public/educators/stc.pdf. Accessed October 2, 2003.

American Association of Directors of Psychiatric Residency Training Psychotherapy Task Force: Psychotherapy competencies. Farmington, CT, American Association of Directors of Psychiatric Residency Training, 2000

American Psychiatric Association: Diagnostic and Statistical Manual of Mental Disorders, 4th Edition, Text Revision. Washington, DC, American Psychiatric Association, 2000

Appelbaum AH, Levy KN: Supportive psychotherapy for borderline patients: a psychoanalytic research perspective. Am J Psychoanal 62:201–202, 2002

Artiss KL: Human behavior under stress: from combat to social psychiatry. Mil Med 128:1011–1015, 1963

Bateman AW, Fonagy P: Effectiveness of psychotherapeutic treatment of personality disorder. Br J Psychiatry 177:138–143, 2000

Beck AT, Sokol L, Clark DA, et al: A crossover study of focused cognitive therapy for panic disorder. Am J Psychiatry 149:778–783, 1992

Beitman B, Yue D: Learning Psychotherapy: A Time-Efficient, Research-Based, and Outcome-Measured Training Program. New York, WW Norton, 1999

Bellack AS, Mueser KT: Psychosocial treatment for schizophrenia. Schizophr Bull 19:317–336, 1993

Bellak L: The schizophrenic syndrome: a further elaboration of the unified theory of schizophrenia, in Schizophrenia: A Review of the Syndrome. New York, Logos, 1958, pp 3–63

Beres D: Ego deviation and the concept of schizophrenia, in The Psychoanalytic Study of the Child, Vol 11. New York, International Universities Press, 1956, pp 164–235

Beutler LE, Moleiro C, Talebi H: Resistance in psychotherapy: what conclusions are supported by research. J Clin Psychol 58:207–217, 2002a

Beutler LE, Moliero CM, Talebi H: Resistance, in Psychotherapy Relationships That Work: Therapist Contributions and Responsiveness to Patients. Edited by Norcross JC. London, Oxford University Press, 2002b, pp 129–143

Birmaher B, Brent DA, Kolko D, et al: Clinical outcome after short-term psychotherapy for adolescents with major depressive disorder. Arch Gen Psychiatry 57:29–36, 2000

Bond M, Banon E, Grenier M: Differential effects of interventions on the therapeutic alliance with patients with personality disorders. J Psychother Pract Res 7:301–318, 1998

Bordin E: The generalizability of the psycho-analytic concept of the working alliance. Psychotherapy: Theory, Research and Practice 16:252–260, 1979

Brent DA, Holder D, Kolko D, et al: A clinical psychotherapy trial for adolescent depression comparing cognitive, family, and supportive treatments. Arch Gen Psychiatry 54:877–885, 1997

Brill L: The treatment of drug abuse: evolution of a perspective. Am J Psychiatry 134:157–160, 1977

Bronheim HE, Fulop G, Kunkel EJ, et al: The Academy of Psychosomatic Medicine practice guidelines for psychiatric consultation in the general medical setting. The Academy of Psychosomatic Medicine. Psychosomatics 39:S8–S30, 1998

Bryant RA, Sackville T, Dang ST, et al: Treating acute stress disorder: an evaluation of cognitive behavior therapy and supportive counseling techniques. Am J Psychiatry 156:1780–1786, 1999

Buckley, P: Supportive therapy: a neglected treatment. Psychiatr Ann 16:515–521, 1986

Busch KA, Fawcett J, Jacobs DG: Clinical correlates of inpatient suicide. J Clin Psychiatry 64:14–19, 2003

Caplan G: An Approach to Community Mental Health. New York, Grune & Stratton, 1961

Carey KB, Coco KM, Simons JS: Concurrent validity of clinicians' ratings of substance abuse among psychiatric outpatients. Psychiatr Serv 47:842–847, 1996

Clark DC, Fawcett J: A review of empirical risk factors for the evaluation of the suicidal patient, in The Assessment, Management, and Treatment of Suicide: Guidelines for Practice. Edited by Bongar B. New York, Oxford University Press, 1992, pp 16–48

Classen C, Butler LD, Koopman C, et al: Supportive expressive group therapy and distress in patients with metastatic breast cancer: a randomized clinical intervention trial. Arch Gen Psychiatry 58:494–501, 2001

Clever SL, Tulsky JA: Dreaded conversations: moving beyond discomfort in patient-physician communication (editorial). J Gen Intern Med 17:884–885, 2002

Cohen DW: Transference and countertransference states in the analysis of pathological narcissism. Psychoanal Rev 89:631–651, 2002

Conte HR: Review of research in supportive psychotherapy: an update. Am J Psychother 48:494–504, 1994

Davanloo H: A method of short-term dynamic psychotherapy, in Short-Term Dynamic Psychotherapy. Edited by Davanloo H. Northvale, NJ, Jason Aronson, 1980, pp 43–71

de Jonghe F, Rijnierse P, Janssen R: The role of support in psychoanalysis. J Am Psychoanal Assoc 40:475–499, 1992

Dewald PA: The strategy of the therapeutic process, in Psychotherapy: A Dynamic Approach. New York, Basic Books, 1964, pp 95–108

Dewald PA: Psychotherapy: A Dynamic Approach, 2nd Edition. New York, Basic Books, 1971

Dewald PA: Principles of supportive psychotherapy. Am J Psychother 48:505–518, 1994

Drake RE, Sederer LI: Inpatient psychosocial treatment of chronic schizophrenia: negative effects and current guidelines. Hosp Community Psychiatry 37:897–901, 1986

Drake RE, McHugo GJ, Noordsy DL: Treatment of alcoholism among schizophrenic outpatients: 4-year outcomes. Am J Psychiatry 150:328–329, 1993

Drake RE, Essock SM, Shaner A, et al: Implementing dual diagnosis services for clients with severe mental illness. Psychiatr Serv 52:469–476, 2001

Dunn C, Deroo L, Rivara FP: The use of brief interventions adapted from motivational interviewing across behavioral domains: a systematic review. Addiction 96:1725–1742, 2001

Elkin I: The NIMH Treatment of Depression Collaborative Research Program: where we began and where we are, in Handbook of Psychotherapy and Behavioral Change. Edited by Bergin AE, Garfield SL. New York, Wiley, 1994, pp 114–139

Elkin I, Shea MT, Watkins JT, et al: National Institute of Mental Health Treatment of Depression Collaborative Research Program. General effectiveness of treatments. Arch Gen Psychiatry 46:971–982, 1989

Epstein RM, Hundert EM: Defining and assessing professional competence. JAMA 287:226–235, 2002

Evans S, Fishman B, Spielman L, et al: Randomized trial of cognitive behavior therapy versus supportive psychotherapy for HIV-related peripheral neuropathic pain. Psychosomatics 44:44–50, 2003

Everly GS Jr, Mitchell JT: Assisting Individuals in Crisis: a Workbook. Ellicott City, MD, International Critical Incident Stress Foundation, Inc., 1998

Everly GS Jr, Mitchell JT: Critical Incident Stress Management (CISM): A New Era and Standard of Care in Crisis Intervention, 2nd Edition. Ellicott City, MD, Chevron Publishing, 1999

Fawcett J, Scheftner WA, Fogg L: Time-related predictors of suicide in major affective disorder. Am J Psychiatry 147:1189–1194, 1990

Fawcett J, Clark DC, Busch KA: Assessing and treating the patient at risk for suicide. Psychiatr Ann 23:244–255, 1993

Fernandez-Pol B, Bluestone H, Mizruchi MS: Inner-city substance abuse patterns: a study of psychiatric inpatients. Am J Drug Alcohol Abuse 14:41–50, 1988

Fischer DE, Halikas JA, Baker JW, et al: Frequency and patterns of drug abuse in psychiatric patients. Dis Nerv Syst 36:550–553, 1975

Foa EB: Trauma and women: course, predictors, and treatment. J Clin Psychiatry 58:25–28, 1997

Foa EB, Franklin ME: Psychotherapies for obsessive compulsive disorder: a review, in Obsessive Compulsive Disorder, 2nd Edition. Edited by Maj M, Sartorius N, Okasha A, et al. Chichester, England, John Wiley, 2002, pp 93–115

Foa EB, Rothbaum BO, Riggs DS, et al: Treatment of posttraumatic stress disorder in rape victims: a comparison between cognitive-behavioral procedures and counseling. J Consult Clin Psychol 59:715–723, 1991

Frank JD: General psychotherapy: the restoration of morale, in American Handbook of Psychiatry, Vol 5: Treatment, 2nd Edition. Edited by Freedman DX, Dyrud JE. New York, Basic Books, 1975, pp 117–132

Freud S: The ego and the id (1923), in The Standard Edition of the Complete Psychological Works of Sigmund Freud, Vol 19. Edited by Strachey J. London, Hogarth Press, 1961, pp 12–66

Freud S: Inhibitions, symptoms and anxiety (1926), in The Standard Edition of the Complete Psychological Works of Sigmund Freud, Vol 20. Edited by Strachey J. London, Hogarth Press, 1959, pp 75–175

Friedman RS, Lister P: The current status of psychodynamic formulation. Psychiatry 50:126–141, 1987

Fudala PJ, Bridge TP, Herbert S, et al, and the Buprenorphine/Naloxone Collaborative Study Group: Office-based treatment of opiate addiction with a sublingual-tablet formulation of buprenorphine and naloxone. N Engl J Med 349:949–958, 2003

Fuller RK, Branchey L, Brightwell DR, et al: Disulfiram treatment of alcoholism: a Veterans Administration cooperative study. JAMA 256:1449–55, 1986

Gabbard GO: A contemporary psychoanalytic model of countertransference. J Clin Psychol 57:983–991, 2001

Galanter M, Castaneda R, Ferman J: Substance abuse among general psychiatric patients: place of presentation, diagnosis, and treatment. Am J Drug Alcohol Abuse 14:211–235, 1988

Gaston L: The concept of the alliance and its role in psychotherapy: theoretical and empirical considerations. Psychotherapy 27:143–153, 1990

Gelso CJ, Fassinger RE, Gomez MJ, et al: Countertransference reactions to lesbian clients: the role of homophobia, counselor gender, and countertransference management. J Couns Psychol 42:356–364, 1995

Gelso CJ, Latts MG, Gomez MJ, et al: Countertransference management and therapy outcome: an initial evaluation. J Clin Psychol 58:861–867, 2002

Gerstley L, McLellan AT, Alterman AI, et al: Ability to form an alliance with the therapist: a possible marker of prognosis for patients with antisocial personality disorder. Am J Psychiatry 146:508–512, 1989

Gill MM, Muslin HL: Early interpretation of transference. J Am Psychoanal Assoc 24:779–794, 1976

Glass A: Psychotherapy in the combat zone. Am J Psychiatry 110:725–731, 1954

Glover E: The therapeutic effect of inexact interpretation: a contribution to the theory of suggestion. Int J Psychoanal 12:397–411, 1931

Glynn SM, Marder SR, Liberman RP, et al: Supplementing clinic-based skills training with manual-based community support sessions: effects on social adjustment of patients with schizophrenia. Am J Psychiatry 159:829–837, 2002

Goldman CR, Quinn FL: Effects of a patient education program in the treatment of schizophrenia. Hosp Community Psychiatry 39:282–286, 1988

Gorton GE: Psychodynamic approaches to the patient. Psychiatr Serv 51:1408–1409, 2000

Greenson RR: The working alliance and the transference neurosis. Psychoanal Q 34:155–181, 1965

Greenson RR: The Technique and Practice of Psychoanalysis. New York, International Universities Press, 1967, pp 190–216

Gunderson JG, Frank AF, Katz HM, et al: Effects of psychotherapy in schizophrenia, II: comparative outcome of two forms of treatment. Schizophr Bull 10:564–598, 1984

Hartley DE, Strupp HH: The therapeutic alliance: its relationship to outcome in brief psychotherapy, in Empirical Studies of Psychoanalytical Theories, Vol 1. Edited by Masling J. Hillsdale, NJ, The Analytic Press, 1983, pp 1–27

Hartmann H: Ego Psychology and the Problem of Adaptation (1939). Translated by Rapaport D. New York, International Universities Press, 1958

Hawton K: Assessment of suicide risk. Br J Psychiatry 150:145–154, 1987

Heinssen RK, Liberman RP, Kopelowicz A: Psychosocial skills training for schizophrenia: lessons from the laboratory. Schizophr Bull 26:21–46, 2000

Hellerstein DJ, Pinsker H, Rosenthal RN, et al: Supportive psychotherapy as the treatment model of choice. J Psychother Pract Res 3:300–306, 1994

Hellerstein DJ, Rosenthal RN, Miner CR: A prospective study of integrated outpatient treatment for substance-abusing schizophrenia patients. Am J Addict 4:33–42, 1995

Hellerstein DJ, Rosenthal RN, Pinsker H, et al: A randomized prospective study comparing supportive and dynamic therapies. Outcome and alliance. J Psychother Pract Res 7:261–271, 1998

Hellerstein DJ, Kocsis JH, Chapman D, et al: Double-blind comparison of sertraline, imipramine, and placebo in the treatment of dysthymia: effects on personality. Am J Psychiatry 157:1436–1444, 2000

Henry WP, Schacht TE, Strupp HH: Structural analysis of social behavior: application to a study of interpersonal process in differential psychotherapeutic outcome. J Consult Clin Psychol 54:27–31, 1986

Henry WP, Schacht TE, Strupp HH: Patient and therapist introject, interpersonal process, and differential psychotherapy outcome. J Consult Clin Psychol 58:768–774, 1990

Ho AP, Tsuang JW, Liberman RP, et al: Achieving effective treatment of patients with chronic psychotic illness and comorbid substance dependence. Am J Psychiatry 156:1765–1770, 1999

Hogarty GE, Kornblith SJ, Greenwald D, et al: Three-year trials of personal therapy among schizophrenia patients living with or independent of family, I: description of study and effects on relapse rates. Am J Psychiatry 154:1504–1513, 1997

Holmes J: Supportive psychotherapy. The search for positive meanings. Br J Psychiatry 167:439–445, 1995

Horowitz M, Marmar C: The therapeutic alliance with difficult patients, in Psychiatry Update: The American Psychiatric Association Annual Review, Vol 4. Edited by Hales RE, Frances AJ. Washington, DC, American Psychiatric Press, 1985, pp 573–585

Horowitz MJ, Marmar C, Weiss DS, et al: Brief psychotherapy of bereavement reactions. The relationship of process to outcome. Arch Gen Psychiatry 41:438–448, 1984

Horvath AO, Symonds BD: Relation between working alliance and outcome in psychotherapy: a meta-analysis. J Couns Psychol 38:139–149, 1991

Hunter J, Leszcz M, McLachlan SA, et al: Psychological stress response in breast cancer. Psychooncology 5:4–14, 1996

Imber SD, Pilkonis PA, Sotsky SM, et al: Mode-specific effects among three treatments for depression. J Consult Clin Psychol 58:352–359, 1990

James RK, Gilliland BE: Crisis Intervention Strategies, 4th Edition. Belmont, CA, Brooks/Cole Thomson Learning, 2001

Jellinek EM: Phases of alcohol addiction. Q J Stud Alcohol 13:673–684, 1952

Kates J, Rockland LH: Supportive psychotherapy of the schizophrenic patient. Am J Psychother 48:543–561, 1994

Kaufman E, Reoux J: Guidelines for the successful psychotherapy of substance abusers. Am J Drug Alcohol Abuse 14:199–209, 1988

Kaufman ER: Countertransference and other mutually interactive aspects of psychotherapy with substance abusers. Am J Addict 1:185–202, 1992

Keller DS, Carroll KM, Nick C, et al: Differential treatment response in alexithymic cocaine abusers: findings from a randomized clinical trial of psychotherapy and pharmacotherapy. Am J Addict 4:234–244, 1995

Kessler RC, McGonagle KA, Zhao S, et al: Lifetime and 12-month prevalence of DSM-III-R psychiatric disorders in the United States: results from the National Comorbidity Study. Arch Gen Psychiatry 51:8–19, 1994

Khantzian EJ: The self-medication hypothesis of addictive disorders: focus on heroin and cocaine dependence. Am J Psychiatry 142:189–198, 1985

Kiesler DJ: Therapist countertransference: in search of common themes and empirical referents. J Clin Psychol 57:1053–1063, 2001

Kleber HD: Pharmacologic treatments for heroin and cocaine dependence. Am J Addict 12 (suppl):S5–S18, 2003

Klein DF, Zitrin CM, Woerner MG, et al: Treatment of phobias, II: behavior therapy and supportive psychotherapy: are there any specific ingredients? Arch Gen Psychiatry 40:139–145, 1983

Kool S, Dekker J, Duijsens IJ, et al: Changes in personality pathology after pharmacotherapy and combined therapy for depressed patients. J Personal Disord 17:60–72, 2003

Koss M, Schiang J: Research on brief psychotherapy, in Handbook of Psychotherapy and Behavior Change. Edited by Bergin A, Garfield S. New York, John Wiley, 1994, pp 664–700

Laikin M, Winston A, McCullough L: Intensive short-term dynamic psychotherapy, in Handbook of Short-Term Dynamic Psychotherapy. Edited by Crits-Christoph P, Barber JP. New York, Basic Books, 1991, pp 80–109

Lamberti JS, Herz MI: Psychotherapy, social skills training, and vocational rehabilitation in schizophrenia, in Contemporary Issues in the Treatment of Schizophrenia. Edited by Shriqui CL, Nasrallah HA. Washington, DC, American Psychiatric Press, 1995, pp 713–734

Lauriello J, Bustillo J, Keith SJ: A critical review of research on psychosocial treatment of schizophrenia. Biol Psychiatry 46:1409–1417, 1999

Lecomte T, Liberman RP, Wallace CJ: Identifying and using reinforcers to enhance the treatment of persons with serious mental illness. Psychiatr Serv 51:1312–1314, 2000

Lehman AF, Herron D, Schwartz RP, et al: Rehabilitation for adults with severe mental illness and substance use disorders: a clinical trial. J Nerv Ment Dis 181:86–90, 1993

Lewis G, Appleby L: Personality disorder: the patients psychiatrists dislike. Br J Psychiatry 153:44–49, 1988

Liberman RP, Wallace CJ, Blackwell G, et al: Skills training versus psychosocial occupational therapy for persons with persistent schizophrenia. Am J Psychiatry 155:1087–1091, 1998

Lindemann E: Symptomatology and management of acute grief. Am J Psychiatry 101:141–148, 1944

Linehan MM: Cognitive-Behavioral Treatment of Borderline Personality Disorder. New York, Guilford, 1993

Linehan MM, Tutek DA, Heard HL, et al: Interpersonal outcome of cognitive behavioral treatment for chronically suicidal borderline patients. Am J Psychiatry 151:1771–1776, 1994

Luborsky L: Principles of Psychoanalytic Psychotherapy: A Manual for Supportive-Expressive Treatment. New York, Basic Books, 1984

Luborsky L, Crits-Christoph P: Understanding Transference: The Core Conflictual Relationship Theme Method. New York, Basic Books, 1990

Malan DH: Individual Psychotherapy and the Science of Psychodynamics. London, Butterworth, 1979

Manring J, Beitman BD, Dewan MJ: Evaluating competence in psychotherapy. Paper presented at the annual meeting of the American Psychiatric Association, San Francisco, CA, May 2003

Markowitz JC, Klerman GL, Clougherty KF, et al: Individual psychotherapies for depressed HIV-positive patients. Am J Psychiatry 152:1504–1509, 1995

Marlatt GA, Gordon JR: Determinants of relapse: implications for the maintenance of behavior change, in Behavioral Medicine: Changing Health Lifestyles. Edited by Davidson PO, Davidson SM. New York, Brunner/Mazel, 1980, pp 410–452

Marlatt GA, Gordon JR: Relapse Prevention: Maintenance Strategies in the Treatment of Addictive Behaviors. New York, Guilford, 1985

Massie MJ, Holland JC: Depression and the cancer patient. J Clin Psychiatry 51 (suppl):12–19, 1990

Menninger K: Theory of Psychoanalytic Technique. London, Imago, 1958

Messer SB: A psychodynamic perspective on resistance in psychotherapy: vive la résistance. J Clin Psychol 58:157–163, 2002

Miller WR, Rollnick S: Motivational Interviewing: Preparing People to Change Addictive Behavior. New York, Guilford, 1991

Misch DA: Basic strategies of dynamic supportive therapy. J Psychother Pract Res 9:173–189, 2000

Mitchell JT, Everly GS Jr: Critical Incident Stress Debriefing (CISD): An Operations Manual for the Prevention of Traumatic Stress Among Emergency Service and Disaster Workers, 2nd Edition. Ellicott City, MD, Chevron Publishing, 1996

Mitchell JT, Everly GS Jr: Critical Incident Stress Management (CISM): Basic Group Crisis Intervention, 3rd Edition. Ellicott City, MD, International Critical Incident Stress Foundation, 2003

Mumford E, Schlesinger HJ, Glass CV: The effect of psychological intervention on recovery from surgery and heart attacks: an analysis of the literature. Am J Public Health 72:141–151, 1982

Novalis PN, Rojcewicz SJ, Peele R: Clinical Manual of Supportive Psychotherapy. Washington, DC, American Psychiatric Press, 1993

Nunberg H: The synthetic function of the ego. Int J Psychoanal 12:123–140, 1931

O'Malley SS, Jaffe AJ, Chang G, et al: Naltrexone and coping skills therapy for alcohol dependence: a controlled study. Arch Gen Psychiatry 49:881–887, 1992

Othmer E, Othmer S: The Clinical Interview Using DSM-IV, Vol 1. Washington, DC, American Psychiatric Press, 1994, pp 87–97

Palmer RL: Dialectical behavior therapy for borderline personality disorder. Advances in Psychiatric Treatment 8:10–16, 2002

Parad HJ, Parad LG: Crisis Intervention, Book 2: The Practitioner's Sourcebook for Brief Therapy. Milwaukee, WI, Family Service America, 1990

Parloff MB: Goals in psychotherapy: mediating and ultimate, in Goals of Psychotherapy. Edited by Mahrer AR. New York, Appleton-Century-Crofts, 1967, pp 5–19

Perry JC, Banon E, Ianni F: Effectiveness of psychotherapy for personality disorders. Am J Psychiatry 156:1312–1321, 1999

Perry S, Cooper AM, Michels R: The psychodynamic formulation: its purpose, structure, and clinical application. Am J Psychiatry 144:543–550, 1987

Persons JB: Cognitive Therapy in Practice: A Case Formulation Approach. New York, WW Norton, 1989

Persons JB: Case conceptualization in cognitive-behavior therapy, in Cognitive Therapies in Action: Evolving Innovative Practice. Edited by Kuehlwein KT, Rosen H. San Francisco, CA, Jossey-Bass, 1993, pp 33–53

Peselow ED, Sanfilipo MP, Fieve RR, et al: Personality traits during depression and after clinical recovery. Br J Psychiatry 164:349–354, 1994

Pine F: The interpretive moment. Variations on classical themes. Bull Menninger Clin 48:54–71, 1984

Pinsker H: A Primer of Supportive Psychotherapy. Hillsdale, NJ, The Analytic Press, 1997

Pinsker H, Rosenthal RN: Beth Israel Medical Center Supportive Psychotherapy Manual (Social and Behavioral Sciences Documents, Vol 18, No 2). New York, Beth Israel Medical Center, 1988

Pinsker H, Rosenthal R, McCullough L: Dynamic supportive psychotherapy, in Handbook of Short-Term Dynamic Psychotherapy. Edited by Crits-Christoph P, Barber JP. New York, Basic Books, 1991, pp 220–247

Pinsker H, Hellerstein DJ, Rosenthal RN, et al: Supportive therapy, common factors and eclecticism. Paper presented at the annual meeting of the American Psychiatric Association, New York, May 1996

Piper WE, Joyce AS, McCallum M, et al: Interpretive and supportive forms of psychotherapy and patient personality variables. J Consult Clin Psychol 66:558–567, 1998

Pokorny AD: Prediction of suicide in psychiatric patients: report of a prospective study. Arch Gen Psychiatry 40:249–257, 1983

Pollack J, Flegenheimer W, Winston A: Brief adaptive psychotherapy, in Handbook of Short-Term Dynamic Psychotherapy. Edited by Crits-Cristoph P, Barber JP. New York, Basic Books, 1991, pp 199–219

Prochaska JO, DiClemente CC: The Transtheoretical Approach: Crossing Traditional Boundaries of Therapy. Homewood, IL, Dow Jones-Irwin, 1984

Psychopathology Committee of the Group for the Advancement of Psychiatry: Reexamination of therapist self-disclosure. Psychiatr Serv 52:1489–1493, 2001

Puryear DA: Helping People in Crisis. San Francisco, CA, Jossey-Bass, 1979

Quality Assurance Project: Treatment outlines for the management of the somatoform disorders. Aust N Z J Psychiatry 19:397–407, 1985

Rea MM, Strachan AM, Goldstein MJ, et al: Changes in coping style following individual and family treatment for schizophrenia. Br J Psychiatry 158:642–647, 1991

Regier DA, Farmer ME, Rae DS, et al: Comorbidity of mental disorders with alcohol and other drug abuse. Results from the Epidemiologic Catchment Area (ECA) study. JAMA 264:2511–2518, 1990

Renaud J, Brent DA, Baugher M, et al: Rapid response to psychosocial treatment for adolescent depression: a two-year follow-up. J Am Acad Child Adolesc Psychiatry 37:1184–1190, 1998

Richard ML, Liskow BI, Perry PJ: Recent psychostimulant use in hospitalized schizophrenics. J Clin Psychiatry 46:79–83, 1985

Robbins B: Under attack: devaluation and the challenge of tolerating the transference. J Psychother Pract Res 9:136–141, 2000

Roberts AR: An overview of crisis theory and crisis intervention, in Crisis Intervention Handbook. Edited by Roberts AR. New York, Oxford University Press, 2000, pp 3–30

Rockland LH: Supportive Therapy: A Psychodynamic Approach. New York, Basic Books, 1989

Rollnick S, Miller WR: What is motivational interviewing? Behavioral and Cognitive Psychotherapy 23:325–334, 1995

Rosenthal RN: Group treatments for schizophrenic substance abusers, in The Group Therapy of Substance Abuse. Edited by Brook DW, Spitz HI. New York, Haworth Medical Press, 2002, pp 329–351

Rosenthal RN, Westreich L: Treatment of persons with dual diagnoses of substance use disorder and other psychological problems, in Addictions: A Comprehensive Guidebook. Edited by McCrady GA, Epstein EE. New York, Oxford University Press, 1999, pp 439–476

Rosenthal RN, Muran JC, Pinsker H, et al: Interpersonal change in brief supportive psychotherapy. J Psychother Pract Res 8:55–63, 1999

Rosenthal RN, Miner CR, Sena P, et al: The therapeutic alliance in group treatments for substance abusers with schizophrenia, in Syllabus and Proceedings Summary, American Psychiatric Association Annual Meeting, Chicago, IL, May 14–19, 2000, Washington, DC, American Psychiatric Association

Rounsaville BJ, Carroll KM: Individual psychotherapy, in Principles of Addiction Medicine. Edited by Graham AW, Schultz TK. Chevy Chase, MD, American Society of Addiction Medicine, 1998, pp 631–652

Safran JD, Muran JC: Negotiating the Therapeutic Alliance: A Relational Treatment Guide. New York, Guilford, 2000, pp 6–12

Salmon TW: War neuroses and their lesson. New York Medical Journal 59:993–994, 1919

Sampson H, Weiss J: Testing hypotheses: the approach of the Mount Zion Psychotherapy Research Group, in The Psychotherapeutic Process: A Research Handbook. Edited by Greenberg LS, Pinsof WM. New York, Guilford, 1986, pp 591–613

Sandoval J: Crisis counseling: conceptualizations and genetic principles. School Psych Rev 14:257–265, 1985

Shear KM, Houck P, Greeno C, et al: Emotion-focused psychotherapy for patients with panic disorder. Am J Psychiatry 158:1993–1998, 2001

Sifneos PE: The prevalence of 'alexithymic' characteristics in psychosomatic patients. Psychother Psychosom 22:255–262, 1973

Sifneos PE: Problems of psychotherapy of patients with alexithymic characteristics and physical disease. Psychother Psychosom 26:65–70, 1975

Simon JC: Criteria for therapist self-disclosure. Am J Psychother 42:404–415, 1988

Skaikeu KA: Crisis Intervention. Boston, Allyn and Bacon, 1990

Smith TE, Hull JW, Goodman M, et al: The relative influences of symptoms, insight, and neurocognition on social adjustment in schizophrenia and schizoaffective disorder. J Nerv Ment Dis 187:102–108, 1999

Spiegel D, Classen C: Acute stress disorders, in Treatments of Psychiatric Disorders, 2nd Edition. Edited by Gabbard G. Washington, DC, American Psychiatric Press, 1995, pp 1521–1536

Stanton AH, Gunderson JG, Knapp PH, et al: Effects of psychotherapy in schizophrenia, I: design and implementation of a controlled study. Schizophr Bull 10:520–563, 1984

Strupp HH, Hadley SW: Specific vs nonspecific factors in psychotherapy. Arch Gen Psychiatry 36:1125–1136, 1979

Sullivan PR: Learning theories and supportive psychotherapy. Am J Psychiatry 128:119–122, 1971

Thomas EM, Weiss SM: Nonpharmacological interventions with chronic cancer pain in adults. Cancer Control 7:157–164, 2000

Thompson LW, Gallagher D: Depression and its treatment. Aging (Milano) 348:14–18, 1985

Tompkins MA: Cognitive-behavioral case formulation: the case of Jim. Journal of Psychotherapy Integration 6:97–105, 1996

Ursano RJ, Silberman EK: Psychoanalysis, psychoanalytic psychotherapy, and supportive psychotherapy, in The American Psychiatric Press Textbook of Psychiatry, 3rd Edition. Edited by Hales RE, Yudofsky SC, Talbott JA. Washington, DC, 1999, pp 1157–1183

Vaillant GE: Adaptation to Life. Boston, MA, Little, Brown, 1977

Vaillant GE (ed): Empirical Studies of Ego Mechanisms of Defense. Washington, DC, American Psychiatric Press, 1986

van Emmerik AAP, Kamphuis JH, Hulsbosch AM, et al: Single session debriefing after psychological trauma: a meta-analysis. Lancet 360:766–771, 2002

Vaughn CE, Leff JP: The influence of family and social factors on the course of psychiatric illness. A comparison of schizophrenic and depressed neurotic patients. Br J Psychiatry 129:125–137, 1976

Volpicelli JR, Alterman AI, Hayashida M, et al: Naltrexone in the treatment of alcohol dependence. Arch Gen Psychiatry 49:876–880, 1992

Wachtel P: Therapeutic Communication: Principles and Effective Practice. New York, Guilford, 1993

Wallerstein RS: Forty-two Lives in Treatment: A Study of Psychoanalysis and Psychotherapy. New York, Guilford, 1986

Wallerstein RS: The psychotherapy research project of the Menninger Foundation: an overview. J Consult Clin Psychol 57:195–205, 1989

Walsh BT, Wilson GT, Loeb K, et al: Medication and psychotherapy in the treatment of bulimia nervosa. Am J Psychiatry 154:523–531, 1997

Waltz J, Addis ME, Koerner K, et al: Testing the integrity of a psychotherapy protocol: assessment of adherence and competence. J Consult Clin Psychol 61:620–630, 1993

Werman DS: The Practice of Supportive Psychotherapy. New York, Brunner/Mazel, 1984

Westerman MA, Foote JP, Winston A: Change in coordination across phases of psychotherapy and outcome: two mechanisms for the role played by patient's contribution to the alliance. J Consult Clin Psychol 24:190–195, 1995

Wilhelm S, Deckersbach T, Coffey B, et al: Habit reversal versus supportive psychotherapy for Tourette's disorder: a randomized controlled trial. Am J Psychiatry 160:1175–1177, 2003

Wilkinson CB, Vera E: Management and treatment of disaster victims. Psychiatr Ann 15:174–184, 1985

Winston A, Winston B: Handbook of Integrated Short-Term Psychotherapy. Washington, DC, American Psychiatric Publishing, 2002

Winston A, Pinsker H, McCullough L: A review of supportive psychotherapy. Hosp Community Psychiatry 37:1105–1114, 1986

Winston A, Rosenthal RN, Muran JC: Supportive psychotherapy, in Handbook of Personality Disorders: Theory, Research, and Treatment. Edited by Livesley WJ. New York, Guilford, 2001, pp 344–358

Woody GE, McLellan AT, Luborsky L, et al: Sociopathy and psychotherapy outcome. Arch Gen Psychiatry 42:1081–1086, 1985

Zetzel ER: Current concepts of transference. Int J Psychoanal 37:369–376, 1956

Ziedonis D, Fisher W: Motivation-based assessment and treatment of substance abuse in patients with schizophrenia. Directions in Psychiatry 16:1–7, 1996

Ziedonis D, Trudeau K: Motivation to quit using substances among individuals with schizophrenia: implications for a motivation-based treatment model. Schizophr Bull 23:229–238, 1997

Zitrin CM, Klein DF, Woerner MG, et al: Behavior therapy, supportive psychotherapy, imipramine, and phobias. Arch Gen Psychiatry 35:307–316, 1978

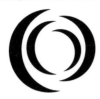

# Index

*Page numbers printed in* **boldface** *type refer to tables or figures.*